'Important and timely. *Breathe, Rest, Recover* is a beacon of hope for anyone battling chronic fatigue or Long Covid. Seamlessly blending yoga wisdom with modern science, this enlightening companion offers clear, compassionate guidance for those looking to heal. A transformative read!'

– Tom Granger, health author and founder of Aria Breath

'The perfect antidote to the (sometimes) reductive tendences of modern medicine, this thoughtful and compassionate book blends evidence-based science with ancient practices in a truly holistic manual. The journey to acceptance or recovery can be a lonely one, and this book will provide those suffering an empathetic and hopeful hand to hold during what can be dark days. It is an invaluable resource for yoga therapists, therapists and healthcare professionals as well as patients experiencing symptoms of Long Covid or any chronic disease. Through practical exercises, we are gently guided in how we might access the tools we have within ourselves to directly influence and heal the inflamed or dysregulated autonomic nervous symptoms, regaining mind-body coherence and allowing for recovery. In the same way that motor and sensory nerves can be rehabilitated after injury, so too can autonomic nerves. The techniques described in this book are accessible, easy to follow and safe.'

– Dr Anna Porter, GP with a special interest in
Long Covid (and lived experience)

'Through personal experience and extensive research, Fiona Agombar and Nadyne McKie offer a resource for hope, inspiration, understanding, support and healing to the millions of people around the world suffering with chronic fatigue, depression and the debilitating effects of Long Covid. They have skilfully tackled what are worldwide epidemics affecting the lives of millions of men, women and even children; reaching all with soothing, understanding and supportive voices; sharing personal experience, extensive research and intelligent and accessible practical guidance towards a return to wellbeing, ease and recovery. In fact, this is a book for everybody in today's stressful world!'

– Simon Low, principal of The Yoga Academy and co-founder of
Triyoga and Santillan Retreat www.simonlow.com

'I loved this book. As ever, Fiona Agombar and Nadyne McKie write clearly and with great compassion. It is accessible for both yoga teachers wanting to support their teaching for all students suffering with fatigue, but also for students themselves, blending scientific evidence with yoga philosophy and ancient teachings. There are several simple practices described, all of which I tried myself and felt great benefits. This is an important and useful book for not only those living with Long Covid but for anyone teaching and living in our fast-paced world.'

– Tamsin Betts, retired GP, yoga teacher, personal
development and career coach

'A powerful piece of literature for the world of yoga therapy! This book beautifully blends science and spirituality, helping the reader to make sense of the complexity of Long Covid, with scientific evidence and theoretical knowledge complimented with gentle accessible yoga therapy practices. The authors thoughtfully address interests of both audiences, encouraging those that struggle with Long Covid to embody practices for recovery, as well as supporting therapists to sensitively expand their understanding and skills in a trauma-informed approach. It is a great contribution both to the academic literature and expanding knowledge base of yoga therapy, but most importantly to the community whom it serves, clients and professionals alike! A fantastic, inspired and informative read, essential for healing from and working with Long Covid!'

– Dr Stephanie Minchin aka The Yoga Psychologist,
founder of House of Yoga Psychology

Breathe, Rest, Recover

by the same author

Yoga Therapy for Stress, Burnout and Chronic Fatigue Syndrome
Fiona Agombar with contributions from Leah Barnett
Foreword by Alex Howard
ISBN 978 1 84819 277 5
eISBN 978 0 85701 223 4

of related interest

Breaking Free from Long Covid
Reclaiming Life and the Things That Matter
Dr Lucy Gahan
ISBN 978 1 83997 350 5
eISBN 978 1 83997 351 2

Mindfulness-Based Therapy for Managing Fatigue
Supporting People with ME/CFS, Fibromyalgia and Long Covid
Fiona McKechnie
Forewords by Rebecca Crane and Dh Taravajra
ISBN 978 1 83997 345 1
eISBN 978 1 83997 346 8

BREATHE, REST, RECOVER

Yoga Therapy for Healing from Long Covid and Fatigue

Fiona Agombar
and **Nadyne McKie**

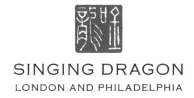

SINGING DRAGON
LONDON AND PHILADELPHIA

First published in Great Britain in 2025 by Singing Dragon,
an imprint of Jessica Kingsley Publishers
Part of John Murray Press

1

Front cover image source: Shutterstock®

A CIP catalogue record for this title is available from the
British Library and the Library of Congress

ISBN 978 1 83997 572 1
eISBN 978 1 83997 573 8

Printed and bound in Great Britain by CPI Group

Jessica Kingsley Publishers' policy is to use papers that are natural, renewable and recyclable
products and made from wood grown in sustainable forests. The logging and manufacturing
processes are expected to conform to the environmental regulations of the country of origin.

Singing Dragon
Carmelite House
50 Victoria Embankment
London EC4Y 0DZ

www.singingdragon.com

John Murray Press
Part of Hodder & Stoughton Limited
An Hachette UK Company

The authorised representative in the EEA is Hachette Ireland, 8 Castlecourt Centre,
Castleknock Road, Castleknock, Dublin 15, D15 YF6A, Ireland

Contents

Acknowledgements

We would like to thank Heather Mason of The Minded Institute who introduced us to each other back in 2021. Thanks to Robin Rothenberg who inspires us with her work, which she shares so generously. Thank you to all the professionals who so kindly endorsed this book. And much gratitude to Claire Wilson, Annie Peacock and Masooma Malik of Singing Dragon for their fantastic support and vision for our book.

NADYNE

Heartfelt gratitude to all my current and previous clients and patients who show great courage in the face of challenge. It's an honour and a privilege to work with you all.

Huge thanks to Dr Edward Douek for his support, guidance and understanding of fatigue-related conditions in children, and to all the doctors and healthcare professionals I meet who refuse to dismiss those experiencing fatigue as people who just need a good nap! My fellow yoga therapists at The Minded Institute, my therapy and counselling buddies and my Priory colleagues who inspire and keep me motivated in so many ways. Dr Anna Walton, Jean-Claude Chalmet and Abigail Iquo Isuo for inspiring and supporting my therapeutic journey. To Tom Granger for allowing me to share his creativity, and to Morgan Scott for the beautiful photographs throughout the book. Thanks to Norman Blair, Dina Cohen, Liz Lark and all my yoga teachers who have inspired me. Special thanks to my family of friends who have supported my work and ridden the rollercoaster of book writing with me. My love and thanks to my son, who inspires me every day and embodies the art of listening to his body with wisdom beyond his years.

And finally, Fiona, a friend for life, who kept me going with coffee, sunshine and inspiration, continually motivating me throughout the journey of writing this book.

FIONA

Thanks to Sarah Ryan, my long-term guide, teacher and friend. I am so glad you are in my life. Thank you for checking the manuscript and the Sanskrit. My mentor, Dr Kausthubah Desikachar, for the amazing insights into the *chakras* and sharing your wisdom on yoga therapy. Vidhi Sadana, yoga therapist and Long Covid pioneer. Jackie Baxter of the Long Covid podcast and Anna Grear of the Fatigue Files podcast, for your inspiring work. Simon Low, thank you. Julia Davies of Yoga Teachers Forum, special thanks for helping to create the Long Covid and ME/CFS online teacher training together with Sarah Ryan. Jyoti Jo Manuel of the Special Yoga Centre and Elizabeth Stanley of Yogacampus who supported my original teacher-training weekends on Stress and ME/CFS. Dr Sarah Myhill, so much gratitude for believing and supporting people like me who live with chronic illness and advocating for us in spite of the challenges. Dr Sam White and Kim Prichard, thank you for your personal support. Dr Tamsin Betts, thank you always. Everyone at the Viniyoga Therapy training in Dorchester, thank you for your love – it is such a privilege to be with you. Thanks to my friend and yogi Leah Barnett for continuing the work and spreading the light. Gratitude to Kathy Martin for explaining why I needed a Virtual Assistant. Dr Joanna Corrado and all the Long Covid team at Leeds Teaching Hospital, thank you for alerting me early on in the pandemic about the help that was needed. Barbara Dancer of the British Council of Yoga Therapy, thank you for putting together the guidelines for those with Long Covid and for introducing me to Suzy Bolt and Nicky Jackson. A special thank you to my Facebook community, Restful Yoga for Fatigue, with Fiona and to everyone there who answered questions and gave the feedback which has helped so much with this book. A special bow of gratitude to all my students, especially the Monday Zoom community. Adyashanti who directed me on my spiritual path, thank you. Special thanks and gratitude to the wonderful Nadyne who is one of the best professionals anyone could wish to work with.

Finally, Thomas Kelly, I couldn't have done it without you.

Introduction

Breathe, Rest, Recover is written for yoga therapists, teachers and healthcare professionals (including nurses, doctors, psychotherapists and counsellors), carers and, of course, those experiencing the chronic symptoms of Long Covid. Because we explore recovery from fatigue, this book is also relevant for those with any form of post-viral fatigue, ME/CFS (Myalgic Encephalomyelitis/Chronic Fatigue Syndrome) and anyone with chronic health problems or breathing pattern disorders.

Our aim is to give the reader a toolbox of practices to promote healing and greater wellbeing through the ancient science of yoga, but that is also informed by contemporary research. We want to empower everyone who reads it, while also considering the constraints and difficulties of modern day living that may impact the potential for recovery.

We both have personal experience of living with and recovering from chronic illness, including severe exhaustion, which is why we know that the tools here work. Because we understand the challenges involved in getting better, we have tried to write clearly, without too much technical jargon. We want to make this book nervous system-friendly and accessible to all, especially those who are experiencing fatigue, brain fog and cognitive dysfunction. Consequently, we encourage you to journey at your own pace.

Take your time. Go gently. Pace. And breathe.

FIONA'S STORY

After a period of intense stress from running a busy PR agency, in 1990 I became very ill with ME (Myalgic Encephalomyelitis), also known as Chronic Fatigue Syndrome (CFS). This lasted for 15 years. I experienced many difficulties, including brain fog and insomnia, but the most distressing symptom was the fluctuating and severe fatigue. This meant that it was almost impossible to engage in everyday life. I eventually made a full recovery, although I had to make many lifestyle changes to do so. This included respecting my stress load – something I continue to honour. So many yoga tools helped that I consequently trained as a teacher and then wrote a couple of books because I wanted to help others with similar experiences. Ultimately, I became interested in yoga as a spiritual path, not just as a healing modality, and I continue to learn from my teachers.

More recently, after a tick bite I developed chronic Lyme disease, which again left me with extreme tiredness. I am now 90 per cent better but still have to pace myself. My feeling is that I became ill a second time because I still had lessons to learn.

With the advent of Covid-19, it became apparent that not everyone was recovering from the virus, and I began to see people in my online classes who had similar symptoms to those of ME/CFS. Over time, this became known as Long Covid. To date, as with ME/CFS, doctors and hospitals are still metaphorically scratching their heads, not knowing what treatment to recommend. Consequently, those with Long Covid may be met with disbelief and lack of empathy. Medical and social gaslighting is still occurring, which we saw for years in the ME/CFS community. In some cases, healthcare professionals will recommend yoga, but all too often their idea is a type of yoga that is inappropriate and may even make someone more unwell or push them into relapse. That's why we knew this book was needed.

In 2021 Heather Mason of The Minded Institute introduced me to psychotherapist and yoga therapist Nadyne McKie. It was the start of a wonderful friendship. I loved Nadyne immediately – she is open, genuine, hugely bright and full of compassion. Nadyne was recovering from Long Covid herself and was learning the hard way, as I had, what worked and what didn't. Her story is told in Chapter 2. Her son also had Long Covid – a challenge for any parent – and Nadyne writes more about this in the final chapter. Nadyne and I agree on so much – that pacing, convalescing and resting are vital, and that our society dismisses chronic illness and pushes us into trying to get active or go back to work too quickly. Ultimately, this can make it much harder to recover, because we have lost the art of convalescence in favour of 'achieve and succeed'. Furthermore, we were both appalled at the level of fear being pushed on mainstream and social media in a way that only serves to heighten nervous system dysfunction and mental health disorders. Potentially, this keeps us in a loop of illness.

We agree that we need to balance *kapha* – an Ayurvedic concept associated with our immunity. This means, from the yoga therapy point of view, that resting after an illness is absolutely vital. And we mean a lot of resting. Nadyne, along with being a respected psychotherapist and yoga therapist, is a science head, whereas I am a yoga geek. She enjoys researching the latest published data while I love the ancient teachings. We hope that you enjoy the mixture that we bring to this book. Because of our mutual health background, we both understand that low-grade chronic stress and trauma impact the nervous system in ways that cause devastation for many of the body's mechanisms. One thing we have learned from the pandemic, for example, is that we need to re-examine how we breathe. Functional breathing is a skill so many of us have lost in Western society, as we whirl faster and faster in our efforts to keep up. Constantly stressed, many of us are breathing too fast, in a way that negatively impacts the whole nervous system. If we then become ill with a virus – the final straw – our chances of a full recovery are severely challenged, particularly if we continue to push on through with a poor breathing pattern. Therefore, addressing the stress response via how we breathe is a priority.

Working with the breath is one of the most important principles of yoga, and part of my own recovery was learning to breathe properly again. *Prana* is the Vedic concept of life force energy, the principle of all energy in the universe. The main connection to *prana* is the breath and the way we direct this. In his wonderful book *The Heart of Yoga*, T.K.V. Desikachar explains that if the out-breath is restricted, ill health is inevitable (Desikachar 1999). Clearly, then, for an illness such as Long Covid, in which 71 per cent claim that fatigue is their most distressing symptom (ONS 2023), *prana* is a very important concept. Indeed, according to yoga, *prana* has the ability to heal most things, if we can utilize it more effectively by undoing 'knots' (called *granthis* in Sanskrit) in our system. It's clear, then, that learning to breathe more functionally encourages profound healing and supports the recovery of health challenges such as Long Covid, if applied together with the other recommendations we share.

Many people with Long Covid have experienced trauma, something else we cover in this book. Consequently, we start by explaining stress and trauma and how to breathe healthily. Throughout the book there are practices, so as you read, you can pause and experience breathing, resting and the peace of yoga for yourself. Yoga is, after all, about the freedom of understanding our true nature, and this comes about with inner peace and a quiet mind. We hope this book will point you towards this.

GUIDANCE FOR FOLLOWING THE PRACTICES IN THIS BOOK

Please read this section before you start any of the practices. You may think of yoga as something that is intense, physical and bendy. Instead, this book explores the tools of yoga therapy, emphasizing quietening and focusing the mind as the foundation for healing on all levels of being. It includes simple, gentle movement, restorative breath practices, relaxation, meditations and optional *mantras*, to soothe and calm the nervous system.

A very important part of yoga is that we want to compassionately observe our more unconscious patterns through self-inquiry, and consequently cultivate new, more positive, habits. We can then bring our new way of being off the mat into our everyday lives. For example, practising regularly helps us to stop and contemplate, process and accept whatever is happening in the present moment. In this way we metabolize stored tension and emotions as well as seeing what is going on in our more unconscious mind. This helps us to reflect and respond, rather than to just react to our experiences in life. We hope that with what follows, you begin to see that the present moment can be a place of great stillness and joy.

NON-VIOLENCE AND SELF-COMPASSION

Another important teaching in yoga therapy is non-violence or, in Sanskrit, *ahimsa*. In the *Yoga Sutras*, *ahimsa* is the first of the *yamas*, or restraints (code of conduct). *Ahimsa* underpins everything we do and always starts with how we treat ourselves and the sense of kindness that we cultivate for our whole being. This also applies to how we practise, so nothing should ever be forced or cause us pain. We need to listen to our bodies so we know when to stop and rest. Then we can take this attitude off the mat and apply it to everything – our planet, our work, how we live and the people we connect with.

A NOTE ON BREATHING PRACTICES

Throughout the book, we give gentle breathing practices to restore health. Some of the more traditional breath practices used in yoga (*pranayama*) are not appropriate for those with Long Covid. *Alternate nostril breathing (unless visualized), anything involving a long breath hold and especially* kapalabhati *(which induces hyperventilation) are contra-indicated for this population. The* ujjayi *breath is also not recommended as it can cause inflammation to the vocal cords.*

There is a misunderstanding that a yogic breath should be full and deep. This is not advisable, and is not the way we teach, as ultimately this can lead to more exhaustion. This is because deep breathing actually creates *less* carbon dioxide, which is needed for oxygen uptake. We explore this more in the breathing chapters, but the general guidance is to breathe 'slow and low' and also through the nose, if possible. Those with Long Covid may have severe breathing problems, so we work towards a better breathing pattern very slowly and gently. In yoga, nothing should ever be forced or uncomfortable, especially the breath. Further guidance is given in Chapters 3, 4 and 5.

FOR ALL THE PRACTICES

As you read, you will find a selection of practices that we have found very helpful for those with Long Covid, ME/CFS and severe fatigue. Remember to modify as required according to symptoms and energy levels, and to practise with kind attention to how you feel on the day at that moment. We offer options and choices with an emphasis on using yoga therapy as a way of exploring what works for you.

Please bear in mind the following:

1. Nothing is compulsory. It's more important that you listen to your body and adapt to what is right for you. We are all here as explorers to discover what works for us as individuals.

2. You will be invited to sit or lie. Make the choice that is right for you. The key word here is to find *comfort*. Find space for your body to breathe and rest. If you are lying, choose the position that feels good. Traditionally, you would lie on your back with your legs extended and slightly apart, arms a little bit away from your body and some support, such as a cushion, under your head. You may, however, be more comfortable with the knees bent or palms on the belly, so experiment

with what feels best. For Long Covid, especially if you have breathing difficulties, you may prefer to lie on your front or side, or to remain seated.

3. Don't force anything. Especially the breath. For some with Long Covid, focusing on the breath can be a source of anxiety. If this is the case, find a different focus for now. This may be on the movements of the belly or the sensation of the hands. In Chapter 2 we guide you to find a Safe Resource, something on which to anchor your attention if you feel anxious or if you are not yet ready to follow the breath.

4. After any breathing practice, rest for a few minutes to let your nervous system restore and recalibrate.

5. Treatment of fatigue must be approached with great respect and caution, as relapse can have serious side effects. Throughout the book, you will find a selection of practices that we have found very helpful for those with Long Covid, ME/CFS and fatigue. However, it's important to remember that this client group are liable to push themselves, and we want to encourage them instead to pace and rest as appropriate.

6. Those with Long Covid are very likely to experience post-exertional malaise (PEM) if there is too much activity. We explain this in more detail in Chapter 11 and in the section on symptoms that follows this. What this means for now is that any practice must be paced according to the individual, and care should be taken not to progress with physical activity too rapidly on higher energy days. We encourage use of the daily check-in, as detailed in Chapter 1, to tune in with awareness. From this, you can learn to listen in and consequently move with how you are, bearing in mind that every day will be different.

7. Chair yoga can be especially useful for those experiencing prolonged fatigue or PEM, as it requires less effort. Most of our practices can be adapted from lying to sitting or vice versa.

8. Yoga therapy empowers you to make good choices that suit you. We are not instructing, but inviting and guiding. We like to think of it as metaphorically holding your hand as you gently travel into a more healing state of being.

9. You may like to record the practices so you can do them without looking at the book and whenever is convenient. When reading out loud, please remember to include lots of pauses and silence. One of the aims is to quieten the mind (fundamental to yogic philosophy) and to calm the nervous system.

10. There is no need to buy specific yoga equipment. Use cushions, blankets, pillows and eye masks as needed, and comfortable, loose clothing. Practise somewhere quiet where you won't be disturbed.

SYMPTOMS OF LONG COVID

There are over 200 symptoms under the umbrella term of 'Long Covid'. Here, we list the main ones:

- *Fatigue, sometimes severe:* This is the most common symptom reported as part of an individual's experience. The severity fluctuates and follows a relapse and remitting pattern. Someone may be full of energy one week, or one day, but then be exhausted or unable to do anything. This means that the yoga practice must always be extremely gentle and not involve too much talking on the part of the teacher, as listening to too much description can increase exhaustion very quickly.

- *Post-exertional malaise (PEM):* This is a really important symptom to understand. PEM refers to the worsening of symptoms following even minor physical or mental exertion. Symptoms typically increase 12 to 48 hours after activity. Individuals may not recognize they have overdone things because it can be challenging to listen to bodily signals communicating fluctuations in energy levels. There is some evidence that the mitochondria (our cells) need time to recover after activity as they can shut down energy function and then take time to restore (Naviaux *et al.* 2016). Too much activity can therefore trigger a relapse. Consequently, all the practices that we give in this book are gentle, with the aim of replenishing *prana*, or energy, to the body.

- *Shortness of breath (dyspnea):* This may be for a number of reasons including damage from the Covid-19 virus to the lungs. Hyperventilation, caused by dysfunctional breathing patterns, chronic stress, trauma and anxiety, is very common. This needs to be addressed gently and with compassion, using the most effective breathing techniques for the individual, while understanding that working with someone with shortness of breath can trigger more anxiety. We therefore explore breathing practices by asking you to go carefully and slowly. You are also strongly advised to avoid some classic yoga *pranayama* exercises, as mentioned.

- *Loss of smell – parosmia and phantosmia:* Parosmia is a condition where sense of smell is distorted. Odours may be perceived as different or unpleasant compared to their usual characteristics, or may not be recognized at all. Individuals with phantosmia may smell scents with no external source causing the odour. These may often be unpleasant. Consequently, if using incense or oils, be aware of this and check in with your client. In yoga philosophy, our sense of smell correlates with the root *chakra (muladhara)*, also associated with a sense of safety and grounding, so we suggest a way of working with scent to induce a feeling of safety in Chapter 2.

- *Brain fog and difficulty concentrating:* Again, this is important to understand because it may be hard to follow instructions. Listening to too much talking can literally hurt the brain. Brain fog also means poor memory, difficulty in interpreting sequences and general cognitive disruption, such as forgetting words and appearing confused.

- *Difficulty sleeping:* Insomnia is very common, which leads to more exhaustion. Deep relaxation practices including yoga *nidra* and rest can help a great deal, as can soothing the nervous system via learning to breathe better.

- *Anxiety and depression (uncertainty, despair, feelings of isolation, fear of the future):* These all feature heavily during illness and recovery, and require empathy and compassion. We suggest working with a yoga therapist or counsellor in addition to following the practices in this book.

- *Heart palpitations:* We advise seeking medical advice before practising the techniques in this book, if heart palpitations are present. This symptom can be very frightening for those with Long Covid, and requires careful monitoring.

- *Chest tightness or pain:* This can also be very frightening and may trigger memories of previous trauma, especially if someone experienced breathing difficulties or heart problems during the acute phase of the illness.

- *Dysautonomia:* This is a disorder of the autonomic nervous system (ANS), affecting heart rate, blood pressure, digestion and temperature regulation. It can lead to symptoms such as dizziness, rapid heartbeat, fatigue and problems with regulating blood pressure.

- *Postural Orthostatic Tachycardia Syndrome (PoTS):* This is a type of dysautonomia characterized by an abnormal increase in heart rate (tachycardia) when transitioning from lying down to standing up. Common symptoms include dizziness, lightheadedness, palpitations, fatigue and nausea. PoTS can also contribute to brain fog. This means we have to be very careful when changing position, and any change of posture should be made very slowly, to allow the heart rate to settle. We explain this more in Chapter 11.

- *Joint or muscle pain:* Known as myalgia and arthralgia, these symptoms involve ongoing discomfort and soreness in muscles and joints, often without an apparent injury or inflammation. Gentle mobilization can reduce discomfort, and we also explore this in Chapter 11.

- *Persistent cough and sore throat:* Vocal cord dysfunction can be part of the Long Covid picture due to chronic coughing and dysfunctional breathing. It's always a good idea to keep warm water to sip nearby and, if lying, to roll onto the front or side. Some people with Long Covid may find lying on their back too uncomfortable, especially if they have a cough, as this can increase breathing problems.

- *Mast Cell Activation Syndrome (MCAS):* This symptom includes an over-activation of histamine, which can cause allergies, so use of incense, perfumes, oils or other allergens may be inappropriate. If you are a therapist, please check with your client.

- *Micro blood clots:* There is some evidence that the primary cause of Long Covid may be micro blood clots, which restrict the flow of blood to the organs and damage the walls of blood vessels. Research is still underway, but this should be considered as it can interfere with oxygen delivery to vital organs affecting functioning of the whole body. This may result in symptoms such as fatigue, brain fog, PoTS, etc. What we offer here in this book is very gentle, so should be of great help.

To conclude, individuals may have some of the above symptoms, or all of them. Some days will be better than others. Some will be severely affected and bed or housebound, whereas others may be able to manage part-time work. In all cases, life will be different from how it was before. In looking at these symptoms, we can understand the need for a unique approach, which is quite different to a general yoga class. This is why yoga therapy is well placed to help support recovery from Long Covid.

Whether you are recovering from Long Covid or fatigue, are a therapist, yoga teacher or health practitioner, we hope what follows will give you plenty of practical tools and ideas on how to work towards healing, and we also hope that you really enjoy the book.

Chapter 1

STRESS: IT'S NOT ALL IN YOUR HEAD

Yoga can be defined as having a peaceful mind, able to focus on the present moment. The mind can be our solution to healing, but it can also be the root of the problem if it is scattered, fearful and chaotic. In the next few chapters, we look at how we can guide the mind to be a quiet refuge and place of rest, rather than something that is filled with worry and anxiety. Our first step is to have a proper understanding of the stress response, so that we can effectively soothe our nervous system in preparation for recovery.

From our experience of working with those with Long Covid, we have found that, in almost all cases, there was a period of chronic stress either before and/or after the initial illness. Many testimonies from clients describe episodes of burnout, stress at work and home, or lives affected by dysfunctional relationships and ongoing family tensions. Because this book is concerned with understanding how we can address the chronic and challenging symptoms of Long Covid, it's essential that we understand the impact of stress on our system and what we can do about it. Self-awareness is a crucial part of this. Ask yourself: 'Is my life stressful for much of the time? Do I know *when* I am actually stressed?' And 'Was I stressed either before or directly after my initial illness, and how did I manage this?' Even if you don't think you have been affected by stress, please read on as you may be surprised. It is possible to be running on overwhelm for so much of the time that it becomes a normal way of being.

LET'S PRACTISE: Checking in (so we don't check out)
This practice is very useful as a daily check-in. When we encounter illness, it's common to feel stuck and disconnected from ourselves. Checking in on a daily basis improves the skill of self-awareness, which is the first step of our healing journey as it allows us to connect to ourselves with curiosity rather than with judgement.

1. Begin by sitting comfortably for a minute or two. If it's okay for you, close your eyes. If this is too much, it's also fine to leave them open. Bear in mind that by closing your

eyes, you support yourself to explore inner awareness. This may take time, so don't judge yourself if you don't want to close your eyes yet.

2. Focus your awareness on the feeling of your body and notice how you are right now. How does it feel to be in this body today? Try not to judge anything – just notice. If there's a story running through your mind, such as 'Oh I feel so tired' or 'I have pain', see if you can be aware of that and also observe yourself being aware, without judgement. If at any time this feels too uncomfortable, bring your focus to your hands and feet.

3. Observe how your mind, body and emotions are right at this moment. Again, try not to have any judgement about your state of being.

4. Can you be aware of your thoughts without trying to still or criticize the mind? Let the thoughts just be there, passing through, like clouds floating by in the sky.

5. How is your energy? Notice any feelings such as tiredness, agitation, anger or sadness. Where do you feel these sensations, for example in your whole body, or your head, or your chest? Again, without judgement, if possible, just notice what's happening. If you can, try to allow everything to be as it is, so that you are doing your best not to resist your current experience. This may seem challenging initially, but remember, all you are doing is practising how to notice, rather than judge. Resistance to your experience is a natural part of exploring awareness.

6. Now, observe the breath. What parts of your body are moving as you breathe? For example, is your chest rising and falling, or maybe your belly? Again, just notice, don't make any assumptions about how this should be. If watching the breath is too much or makes you feel agitated in any way, come back to feeling your hands and feet.

7. Slow the breath down a little if you are able to. Place one hand on the heart and one on the belly and see if you can breathe into the hand at your belly, keeping the hand on the heart space relatively still. If you can't do this, that's fine too.

8. Take five slightly slower breaths. This isn't about breathing deeply – think of the breath being slow and low. For some people with Long Covid, watching the breath or trying to alter it in any way can increase anxiety, so if this is you, just observe the movement of your body beneath your hands, or leave this bit out for now.

9. Now return to normal breathing, again noticing how you are right now.

10. Are there any changes to how you feel? However slight these are, allow yourself to just be aware. Again, try not to judge, and see if you can just be curious.

11. Bring your attention to your thoughts. Are your thoughts fast or slow? Is the mind darting about or is there a sense of stillness? Without any judgement, notice your mind.

12. Bring your awareness to your feet and hands, making small movements with the fingers and toes. Now come back to the body and move a little.

13. Open your eyes if they are closed. Sit for a moment or two and look around your space, feeling yourself here, in this moment. Slowly ease yourself back into your day.

WHAT HAPPENS WHEN WE ARE STRESSED

Stress is both a physiological and psychological response to a perceived threat or demand. We are wired to fight, flight or freeze if we think there is danger, just like our ancestors who had to deal with life or death situations every day. In these modern times, stress is more likely to be caused by a variety of factors such as work, finances, relationships, health…or a chronic illness. When we believe that we are under threat, our sympathetic nervous system (SNS) immediately fires up the stress response, also known as the fight or flight response. This releases hormones such as cortisol and adrenaline, which have multiple effects on our system, including increasing our heart and breathing rate and raising blood pressure. Blood then drains from our major organs to our limbs, which helps us to either run fast from danger or to stay and fight. This is fine if there is an actual threat, such as if we are being attacked, but most of the time, the stress we encounter isn't life threatening. Once the perceived threat has passed (and note, we say 'perceived' because stress is very much to do with our perception of a situation), then the parasympathetic nervous system (PNS) kicks in to help our hormone levels return to normal. The heart rate consequently decreases and blood pressure returns to its baseline.

The PNS is also known as the 'rest and digest' division, and during this phase, you may feel quite tired, achy and foggy while the body heals. If you are used to being chronically activated, you may even feel bored, because being aroused from low-level stress can be addictive. Think of scrolling through social media, which triggers certain chemicals such as dopamine. This is associated with the reward circuit of the brain and keeps us scrolling in anticipation of finding something beneficial. However, it's very important to rest after a period of stress, and to not keep going, otherwise the healing process can't happen because the nervous system is unable to regulate and dial down activation. If our system is unable to properly recover, we may find ourselves stuck in a high alert pattern with tense muscles, fast, shallow breathing, and a chronically raised heart rate, all of which affect the immune system. You might not be conscious of this happening, which is why we emphasize self-awareness a great deal. In this book, we repeat the importance of proper rest and convalescence because of the need to let the stress chemicals discharge so that our system can recover. Resting also helps our mitochondria (the energy cells of the body) to restore so that they don't go into shutdown mode. There's more on the importance of the mitochondria in Chapter 3.

The key system for regulating the body's stress response is called the hypothalamic-pituitary-adrenal (or HPA) axis. The hypothalamus is a crucial area of the brain centre, working to keep our body in a state of homeostasis, or healthful balance. The HPA axis enables the body to adapt to stressors through the release of stress hormones, such as cortisol. Cortisol helps the body cope with stress by increasing blood sugar levels, enhancing alertness and suppressing the immune system. All this is vital for survival. However, long-term activation of the HPA axis has negative effects on our nervous system and can lead to dysregulation and imbalances in the body, contributing to various health problems such as impaired immune function, auto-immune disorders, anxiety and depression.

We need small amounts of stress in order to survive. Hormesis, for example, describes how short-term bursts of stress, such as exposure to very cold or hot temperatures, and certain breathing techniques, can make us more resilient. When we are unwell, however, applying a hormetic stressor is unwise, and is likely to make us even more fatigued. For example, cold water plunges would not be advisable for most people with Long Covid.

THE ROLE OF INFLAMMATION

Inflammation is a key response to defend us against illness and stress. When we are running a chronic stress response over a long period of time, our bodies switch on the inflammatory process to protect and heal the body. However, chronic and excessive inflammation can impair the healing process by dysregulating the immune system and increasing susceptibility to illness and infection. To add to the picture, when we are unwell, we often feel low in mood. The elevated inflammatory response contributes to creating these feelings, which is why we may notice we feel down when we are sick. If we are in tune with our bodies and aware of this, we can sense these feelings are just a reaction to being ill. This can guide us to look after ourselves better by eating more nourishing food and by resting. We may find stopping and resting difficult, however, and we look at why this is later on.

BUT I AM NOT STRESSED!

Chronic stress is often so low grade that there may be little awareness of it happening. There may be a vague feeling of being hyperaroused, as if there is too much caffeine coursing through the system. Other symptoms include finding it difficult to switch off or relax, feeling anxious, bouts of insomnia, low mood, frequent bursts of irritation, feeling less empathetic to those around us, finding it difficult to make decisions, digestion problems including Irritable Bowel Syndrome (IBS), aches and pains from tense muscles, exhaustion, feeling tired but wired and a feeling that life is frequently overwhelming and unmanageable.

Someone with constant stress may feel dissociated from their body, or conversely, hyperaware of any physical function such as a raised heartbeat. The common way of coping with this discomfort is to add in more activities to keep busy and distracted, such as watching TV, overworking, shopping or scrolling through social media in order to take away any emotional pain or unpleasant symptoms. In other words, anything rather than rest. We may even use yoga as a distraction, forcing our bodies into shapes we think we 'should' make. This can be especially the case if we are going to stronger *vinyasa* classes because we mistakenly think exercise is the answer. We may also use stimulants to self-soothe, such as coffee, alcohol or sugar, or excessive exercise, all of which may temporarily help, but ultimately make our health worse. These strategies, although encouraged by our culture, actually play havoc with our nervous system, keeping us in a state of sympathetic activation.

THE STRESS–BREATH–FEAR CYCLE

When we are stressed, the breath speeds up in order to prepare the system to run, or to stay and fight. As we breathe faster, however, our mind responds by thinking more quickly. This is a survival mechanism that is needed to get us out of danger fast. However, if we are chronically stressed, our thoughts typically become faster and more anxious. We may focus on our symptoms, which increases our anxiety even more. This, in turn, makes us breathe more quickly, perpetuating a stress response. We are then locked into a cycle of fearful, speedy thinking, symptom focusing and fear, more rapid breathing and then further, chronic activation. The way out of this is to breathe more healthfully – something we examine in later chapters.

LET'S PRACTISE: The physiological sigh

This breathing technique has shown evidence of greater improvement in mood, increased reduction in anxiety and reduction in the respiratory and heart rate, which we know has an impact on calming our stress response. Research shows that physiological sighs improve brain function, allowing an individual to experience joy, calm and focus, more so than mindfulness meditation (Balban *et al.* 2023). We want to highlight that although sighing can be helpful for immediate short-term relief when used as a specific practice, excessive sighing as a habitual response can exacerbate fatigue and anxiety due to hyperventilation. So, use the following practice just once or twice a day, if you are feeling anxious.

1. Sit comfortably and feel your feet in contact with the ground.

2. Bring attention to your breath. Inhale slowly through the nose, if you can, and then take another slightly longer 'top-up' inhale, like an extra sniff of air.

3. Slowly exhale out all the breath by sighing out through the mouth. Ideally, the two inhalations are through the nose, then you exhale with a sigh.

4. Repeat this a few times to get familiar with the practice.

5. Over time you can build up to five rounds of two inhalations, followed by a sigh.

CHRONIC STRESS AND LONG COVID

When it comes to Long Covid, stress will obviously exacerbate symptoms and delay recovery. The conundrum is, of course, that having a chronic illness that impacts the work–life balance is in itself stressful. It's not all bad news, however, and we are not trying to incite fear by explaining how damaging stress is. The point is that we *can* learn to manage the stress response with many of the soothing yoga techniques that are in this book. However, it's important that you understand what stress means *for you*, and that you get a feeling for when you are stressed and when you are not. Tuning in to how you feel with awareness, as described in the first practice, will help you to recognize when you actually are experiencing stress, so you can then take action to change the state of your nervous system. We give you tools for this later on.

Emma[1] was in a job she disliked, working long hours and not feeling particularly fulfilled when she caught Covid. She was also supporting her partner, a recovering alcoholic, who had relapsed during the pandemic, so she found it difficult to take the rest that was needed. She found it hard to seek support or acknowledge her stress load. She experienced debilitating fatigue and moved back to her parents' house, to convalesce. During her recovery, and thanks to yoga and breathing practices, she was able to understand how stress was impacting her health and adding to her cycles of push–crash–relapse. She consequently decided to end the relationship with her partner and is now retraining as a gardener, something she always longed to do.

LET'S PRACTISE: Rocking to soothe

The gentle rhythmical rock of a rocking chair...the soothing rocking of a baby...a hammock swaying slowly in the breeze... Rocking our bodies is a tried and tested practice to soothe and engage the PNS. Restorative rocking helps to regulate our nervous system, improving sleep, memory and focus, inducing a sense of calm. The motion of rocking synchronizes

---

1   All names in the book have been anonymized.

the brain and increases our ability to sleep through environmental noise (Bayer *et al.* 2011). Rocking and the accompanying soothing of the nervous system encourages us to slow down, and promotes a sense of safety in the body.

1. You may wish to try rocking in various positions, so experiment with lying, sitting, standing or on your belly.

2. Here, we guide you from a lying position, perhaps on your right side with cushioned support under any parts of your body that need it. You may wish to hug a pillow to your belly and support your head with a cushion. Alternatively, sit in a comfortable, supported position.

3. Invite an awareness of your body. Notice the parts in contact with the ground.

4. Begin to rock or sway gently, side to side, or back and forth, in a gentle rocking motion. If you are on your side, take the top hand level with the belly and push on the hand to rock. You can explore how you rock – small or large movements, faster or slower.

5. If seated, it can feel soothing to place your arms around yourself across the shoulders, but allow this to be gentle and not too tight.

6. If you are on your back, invite the movement to begin from the feet upwards, allowing the body to move gently into rhythmic rocking.

7. Continue to sway and rock, focusing on the rhythm of the rocking.

8. If you have a rocking chair or swing or hammock, you can also try using this to explore this movement.

THE ROLE OF THE PANDEMIC ON STRESS LEVELS

Stress levels increase when there is lack of social connection, a feeling of being unsafe and uncertain, and a perception of loss of control. All three were dominating factors throughout the Covid crisis, affecting us both physically and emotionally. It's obvious with hindsight how the pandemic increased global anxiety in so many ways – closures of schools and universities, financial uncertainty, social isolation, fear of infecting vulnerable family members, health anxiety – the list goes on. The message from the media was one of misinformation, mistrust and fear. We were told to be afraid. But when we don't know who to trust, our very foundations are shaken. We lose our inner sense of security, and begin to doubt that the world is safe and reliable. Significantly, lockdown meant avoidance of other people to prevent infection. For many, this created a sense of isolation from our communities, friends and loved ones. Unfortunately, these fear messages continue as we are bombarded with news of potential climate disaster, geopolitical tensions, the threat of new viruses and social polarization around many issues.

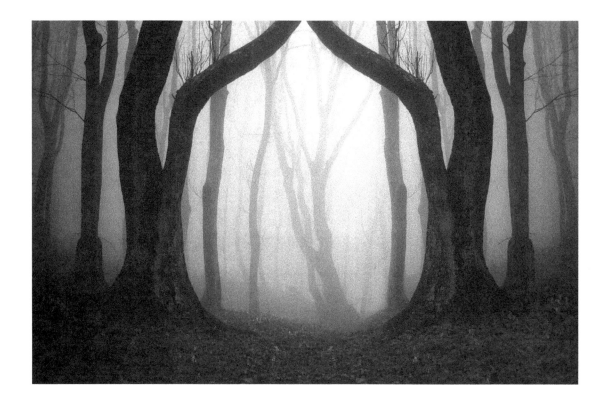

When we are afraid, angry and anxious, we are kept in the 'doing' rather than 'being' state and our nervous system becomes chronically dysregulated. In essence, we collectively experience the trauma of living in an uncertain world. This may manifest in unhealthy coping mechanisms, such as the distractions we explained previously and which are used to avoid underlying emotions such as fear, isolation and tension. Addressing this involves awareness and acceptance of our physical and mental symptoms as they arise in each moment, and the ability to meet difficult feelings with self-compassion and kindness. In other words, if we can gradually learn how to stay present and tolerate our more demanding emotions rather than distracting ourselves by keeping busy and pushing through, we can better manage and discharge any stress, which, in turn, means the body can start to heal.

Regulation of the nervous system is, after all, the foundation of health and wellbeing. Therefore, to heal we must firstly address nervous system dysregulation. All the practices that we share address nervous system recovery via soothing and gentle movement, functional breathing and nourishing, and restorative rest.

When we practise yoga, we can explore our sensations with curiosity. As we become more aware, this reveals our ways of operating that may hinder the healing process. For example, Mary had a habit of constantly checking things online in order to distract herself from her anxiety of Covid reinfection. All the screentime, however, made her more exhausted, and the endless information she was reading, especially about the world news, just increased her stress load. As her yoga practice developed, she realized how unhelpful this was to her recovery, and she was able to reduce her screentime and use yoga tools that helped to bring more calmness and resilience into her daily life.

PHYSICAL SIGNS OF STRESS

- Clenched jaw

- Hunched, raised shoulders

- Fast breathing, sometimes from the mouth, with the chest rising up and down quickly

- Speaking fast

- Disconnected from Self and others, and detached from the surrounding environment

- Muscle tension

- Poor eye contact, darting eyes

- Finding it difficult to be still or in the present

- Difficulty speaking, or remembering words

- Agitation and impatience – we may see students or clients rushing through postures in a yoga class

- Body posture with chest collapsed and head dropped.

SOCIAL CONNECTION AND CO-REGULATION

An important antidote to stress is *co-regulation*. This means a safe connection to a calm and trusted other person. When we are with someone we trust and who makes us feel secure, this dials down activation from the stress response. A dog, cat or other pet can also give emotional support and help to soothe during times of distress. Co-regulation can be greatly helped by a yoga teacher or therapist, *providing they are able to effectively self-regulate their own nervous system and are fully present for the student*. In other words, the therapist must offer the same compassion, kindness and non-judgement to themselves that they are encouraging in others. Otherwise, the therapist may actually contribute to the dysregulation of those they are working with.

CO-REGULATION AND SAFETY: THE ROLE OF THE TEACHER OR THERAPIST

From the yogic perspective, the concept of connection and safety is essential to alleviate suffering and stress. In yoga therapy, great emphasis is therefore placed on coming from the heart to cultivate an authentic, non-judgemental relationship with the client. This is particularly relevant for individuals post-Covid, who may be experiencing symptoms of stress, trauma and anxiety in addition to feeling judged and misunderstood, especially if they have experienced medical gaslighting (Outhoff 2020). Stephen Porges' Polyvagal Theory (PVT) (explained further in Chapter 2) emphasizes the need for the creation of a safe space and safe 'other' in order to down-regulate and soothe the nervous system: 'The real issue in therapeutic relationships is whether the individual is safe in the presence of the other' (Geller and Porges 2014). In other words, if you are a yoga teacher or therapist, it's not just about applying yoga tools; it is also about the relationship you create with your student, and how you can help them to feel safe and supported. In yoga therapy, a heart-based relationship is considered fundamental, because it creates the foundation of safety necessary for healing. Empathy, authenticity, unconditional positive regard and non-judgement are essential traits of an effective yoga therapist. We can employ certain techniques to assist this process, such as deep, active listening, warmth, openness and eye contact, and via use of an authentic caring voice. But the most important quality is the ability to hold a secure space and demonstrate genuine compassion so that the client feels that they are safe enough to be vulnerable.

CULTIVATING CONGRUENCE

Language conveys energy and words hold great power. We know that the tone of our voice and facial expressions indicate meaning without words. Therefore, our use of language needs to be carefully considered, and we should aim to use invitational guidance, rather than instructing or dictating how things 'should' be done or look. Language can communicate either compassion or rigidity, and we should move away from goal-oriented practices towards exploration. In other words, there is no right way of doing yoga. So, we might use phrases like 'open' rather than 'stretch' and 'explore' rather than 'reach'. 'Allow', 'release', 'ease', 'soften', 'notice', 'investigate' and 'be curious' are other examples of words or phrases that encourage the student to feel rather than to think, or over-analyse, what is happening. In this way, we take the student out of their head and more into their body and feelings, thus promoting a safe space in which they can explore their whole being with curiosity and self-compassion, away from the realms of judgement.

This is a major step in guiding someone out of the stress response and encouraging a healing state. As teachers and therapists, it requires that we come from a place of our own internal sense of safety, so it is important that we are doing our own self-inquiry and daily practice too. Are we calm, for example, or are we in sympathetic overdrive and stressed before we teach? This might sound obvious, but yoga teachers get anxious and burnt out too! Ultimately, we are helping those with Long Covid to become more embodied, more self-aware and more accepting of their current situation by letting them know they are safe and supported. This in itself will dramatically help to reduce stress and promote recovery.

OTHER WAYS YOGA CAN HELP

As we have seen, creating safety is an important remedy to the stress response because a feeling of being secure affects our whole nervous system, including our breathing. When we breathe effectively, our PNS takes over and we increase the healthy function of our vagus nerve, which connects the brain and the gut (we explain this in more detail in the next chapter). There are many techniques that we share in this book to help with this process. One of the most important is functional breathing, which we explain in Chapters 3, 4 and 5. Healthy breathing is vital because breathing dysfunctionally keeps us locked in a chronic stress pattern. Learning to breathe well is the ultimate bio-hack in soothing the stress response.

EXPLORING ACTIVATION

In order to change how we perceive threats, we have to give our body the space and time to slowly, gently and safely explore the smallest amount of activation that arises around challenges. Even just being present in the body for the first time during a yoga practice can seem threatening for some, because there may be a new awareness of unpleasant symptoms. Dissociation is no longer possible. Yoga, however, is a great way to begin this exploration, if applied appropriately, and there are lots of tools later on, such as gentle movement to mobilize the spine and diaphragm, deep rest and working with the *chakras* or energy centres. All of these can make a profound difference to recovery. Completely avoiding stress, after all, is not possible, and trying to think our way out of stress doesn't really work either. Telling ourselves that we are 'fine' can lead to further disconnection from our bodies so that we bypass our alarm system. Our stress response and its effect on the body therefore needs to be acknowledged. Yoga helps with this connection and puts us back in the driving seat.

LET'S PRACTISE: Humming and moving mindfully

This practice incorporates breathing with a very gentle moving sequence.

1. From a comfortable sitting position, become aware of your body. Take a moment or two to notice the parts in contact with your support, such as your bottom on the chair or feet on the floor.

2. Welcome yourself, however you are right now. Relax your jaw. Relax your eyes. If it's comfortable for you, you might like to close your eyes.

3. Think about your posture and how you are sitting. See if you can create more space between your tailbone and crown of the head. Let your lower ribs softly open as you slightly lift your heart, so there is an alertness but no strain in the way you are sitting.

4. Observe your mind, your physical body and your emotions. Can you allow everything to be just as it is at this moment? Can you bring acceptance to this moment or even kindness to your state of being – even if there is fatigue or pain? Take a moment or two to gather compassion for yourself, just as you are, here in this moment. If at any time you feel anxious, bring your awareness back to the feeling of your body in contact with your support and a sense of solidity holding you.

5. If you are comfortable following the breath, observe your breathing for a moment or two. Begin to slow your breathing down slightly to a comfortable rhythm. You might like to visualize that you are breathing in a sense of safety into the heart on the in-breath, then releasing and letting go on the out-breath. If you are not okay with following the breath, or not yet ready to work with the concept of safety, just feel the small movements in your body as your breath changes.

6. For the next five breaths (always remembering that everything is optional – you could do this for just one or two breaths), hum the breath out slowly on the exhalation, by bringing the lips together and sounding a hum of one note.

7. We are going to add some movement, so start with your hands on your knees. Inhale and gently float your arms up in front of you and then above your head, or to wherever is comfortable, in time with the in-breath. As you exhale, again hum and bring the arms down, finishing with the hands on the knees at the end of the exhalation, so the movement is in time with the humming. Repeat up to five times.

8. Pause, and observe the effect of the humming on the whole system. Be curious. Explore how you are now – mind, body, emotions and breath.

9. Continue to breathe slowly if it feels okay, but it's also fine if you can't do this today. If you can, just take a moment or two to focus on each exhalation, seeing if you can make the out-breath long and smooth. Now, if you would like to, come down to lying. It's also fine to remain sitting if that's better for your breathing. If you are on your back, have your knees bent, feet hip width apart and maybe some support under your head. You can gently bring the knees together to touch each other if you are very fatigued.

10. Touch the floor or your support with your hands, exploring how this feels, and become aware of your connection with this support. If you are on a chair, you can explore the sensation of the floor under your feet.

11. On every exhalation, relax and release into your support. Imagine that you are lying (or sitting) on a warm beach, on slightly damp sand. On every out-breath, as your body becomes more relaxed, you become heavier, so the indentation of your body is making a shape in the warm sand. Feel your body and the sand merging together.

12. On your in-breath, focus on breathing in peace. If you like, you can chant 'Shanti' on every exhalation for a few breaths. This is a Sanskrit word which means peace. This is a choice – you don't have to chant if you don't want to. It's also fine to chant in English – you can use 'Peace'. Pause after a few breaths and focus on the sensation or idea of peace.

13. Take a moment to feel what peace means for you. Inner peace is important and is something that we take time to cultivate, perhaps by being still a few times a day, perhaps by taking micro-breaks whenever possible. It's a very precious commodity to nurture.

14. If you have no back issues (and if you are on your back), straighten out your legs, having the heels comfortably apart.

15. Inhaling, let the arms float up wide and behind you. The back of your hands might touch the floor, but if they don't, have the arms wider apart or place a cushion behind your head to support the arms and hands. As you exhale, bring the arms back beside the body with the palms turned down beside the hips. If you like, you can chant 'Shanti' or 'Peace' slowly as the arms travel back on the out-breath. If you don't want to chant, you can hum or just breathe out slowly, in time with the movement.

16. Repeat this 3–5 times, as if it is a moving meditation with the mind, breath, sound and movement all as one. Just focus on the slow movement and the breath.

17. Now pause and see how you feel. Take a moment to observe your body, mind and emotions, allowing everything to be as it is. Drop this reflective statement into the silence: 'I am enough.' How does this statement make you feel? Just explore your state of being with curiosity and non-judgement.

THE IMPORTANCE OF GROUNDING

One of the most effective ways that we can develop a sense of safety in yoga is to use a grounding practice. We do this by feeling the connection with the feet to the floor or our back with its support, such as a mat, chair or bed. The benefits of grounding are increased if we practise outside in nature because then we feel the actual earth beneath our feet, and remind ourselves of our connection to the planet and nature around us. If you can, spend some time each day outside, reminding yourself to look up at the sky, as so much of our time is spent looking down at screens. Walking barefoot outside is also a great practice. Being in nature calms the system and allows us to recentre and replenish.

One of the advantages is that walking outside encourages us to move the eyes laterally. This has the benefit of down-regulating the fear centre of the brain (the amygdala). Our sense of grounding and of being here as part of the world is also about our root *chakra* (*muladhara*), and we explore this more later. If you are too unwell to go outside, you may like to open a window and look at the sky or visualize being in nature.

LET'S PRACTISE: Grounding

1. Find an easeful posture that works for you. This could be sitting, or lying with knees bent.

2. Begin by feeling your feet in contact with the floor. Bring awareness to your breath. Allow yourself to follow the journey of the breath as you slowly inhale and exhale. If following the breath makes you feel anxious, think of something that makes you feel safe – this might be a loved one, a pet, a place in nature or feeling into the softness of your hands. Just focus on the image of this as your Safe Resource.

3. Take time to adjust your breathing rhythm, gently drawing each breath lower into the body, allowing the belly to rise and fall slightly with each inhale and exhale. Think of the breath as being low rather than being too deep.

4. Connecting to our senses encourages us to be in the present moment, finding safety and calm in the environment around us. So, take time now to identify the following:

   - 5 things you can see

   - 4 things you can touch

   - 3 things you can hear

   - 2 things you can smell

   - 1 thing you can taste.

5. Inwardly name these things, taking time to allow for slow, gentle breathing.

6. Place one hand on your lower belly. Feel the sensation of the rise and fall with each breath.

7. Again, feel your feet in contact with the floor. Focus on the sensation under your feet. What texture can you feel? Can you feel warmth or coolness? Are there any sensations in the soles of the feet? Any vibration?

8. Begin to wriggle your toes, your fingers, and slowly, with care, ease yourself back into the day.

WORKING WITH, NOT AGAINST, THE NERVOUS SYSTEM

In writing this book, we are aware that we have included many practices. When we are unwell, there is often a drive to do as much as possible in order to heal. It's important to remember, however, that to get better, we need to rest and respond more kindly to our body, perhaps in ways that we have ignored for many years. This takes time. Our suggestion is to make small changes, slowly. Allow the nervous system to adjust gradually. In other words, don't rush through all the practices at once – just pick one or two that you'd like to start with. Another way we encourage this idea of slowing down is to adopt lots of small micro-breathing breaks into your day (more on that in Chapter 3).

In the next chapter we look at why it may be more challenging to recover from Long Covid if there is a history of trauma, and how to approach healing from a place of awareness and self-compassion.

KEY POINTS

✓ The mind can help us in our recovery, or it can be a barrier to getting better. Yoga helps it to be the former.

✓ Understanding how the stress response works can help us to heal.

✓ Checking in with how we are daily helps us to improve the important skill of self-awareness.

✓ When we are stressed, the sympathetic nervous system (SNS) produces certain hormones, which fires up the fight or flight response.

✓ When the stress has passed, the parasympathetic nervous system (PNS) should bring the body back to normal. We may feel tired and achy while this happens as the system is being repaired.

✓ If we are continuously activated, we may be running a low-level stress response. Over time, this will damage our system and cause chronic inflammation.

✓ We may not be aware that we are stressed, even though we may have unpleasant symptoms including tension, anxiety, poor posture and a feeling of not being safe. A common way to deal with this is to keep busy and distracted.

✓ When we are stressed, we breathe faster, maybe from the chest and through the mouth. This can keep us chronically activated.

✓ Helpful tools from yoga include rocking, breathing and sighing to soothe the nervous system. Grounding is also important, which we can do with an appropriate yoga practice.

✓ Social connection and co-regulation with a trusted 'other' such as a yoga therapist can quickly reduce a chronic stress response and helps to make us feel safe.

✓ It is very important that the yoga therapist takes time for their own practice in order to be regulated, authentic and compassionate.

Chapter 2

TRAUMA: HOW THE PAST IMPACTS HEALTH

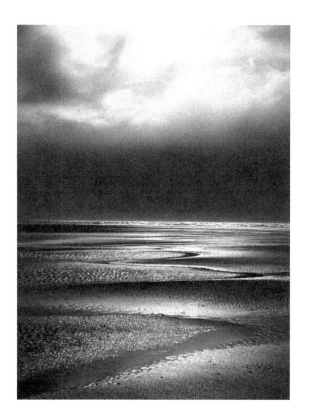

When we began working with people with Long Covid, we noticed a striking similarity when taking their past health and life history: many had experienced significant trauma. Trauma describes any experience that overwhelms our ability to cope, to the extent that the body is unable to effectively process what has happened. Trauma can result from various life situations. What is traumatic to one may not be to another. Trauma is subjective and depends on a number of factors, such as childhood experiences, early attachment to caregivers, and the impact on the nervous system. Therefore, each person's individual response to a situation should always be respected and never judged or doubted.

Whether a person experiences a one-off traumatic event or a series of ongoing stressful situations, the body's stress response is activated, leading to the release of certain hormones. In normal circumstances, as we saw in the previous chapter, these help the body prepare for the stress response by mobilizing energy and increasing alertness. After the stress has passed, the central nervous system (CNS) should come back to a state of homeostasis. However, in cases of trauma, the CNS can become chronically dysregulated. When stress hormones are continuously elevated, they can become trapped or stored within the CNS. The body's natural mechanisms for processing them may then become overwhelmed or disrupted, preventing efficient clearance. If we are then reminded of a traumatic event, we may experience this as a 'trigger', which prompts the body to experience the trauma reaction again, even if this is not relevant to what is currently happening. We may then become hyper- or hypoaroused when provoked, meaning that we either become highly anxious and agitated, or we shut down and dissociate from our current experience. More commonly, we may swing between these two states.

HOW DOES THE PAST IMPACT THE PRESENT?

If you had a childhood that was chaotic or disruptive, you may be more sensitive to the effects of trauma. Traumatic events during childhood are known as Adverse Childhood Experiences (ACEs), a term first coined by Vincent Felitti in 1998 (Felitti *et al*. 1998). Examples of ACEs include domestic violence, abuse, divorce, growing up in a family with mental illness, substance misuse issues, or feeling unloved during childhood. Chronic stress resulting from ACEs can alter brain development and affects how the body responds to stress later in life. According to one study, individuals who had experienced two or more early traumatic events were 5.6 times more likely to exhibit symptoms of Long Covid (Van Den Hurk *et al*. 2022). Research demonstrates that exposure to childhood trauma was associated with a six-fold increased risk of developing CFS (Heim *et al*. 2009). We want to make it clear that we are not trying to pin Long Covid or CFS as a trauma response, but we are suggesting that trauma may be part of the picture that needs addressing, in order to support recovery.

SYMPTOMS OF POST-TRAUMATIC STRESS DISORDER

When we talk about trauma in this chapter, we also mean Post-Traumatic Stress Disorder (PTSD), and complex PTSD, or C-PTSD. C-PTSD is a condition that develops after experiencing long-term trauma, often related to the developmental years or ongoing abuse, and includes additional symptoms such as difficulties with emotional regulation, social connection, dissociation, hyper-vigilance and feelings of worthlessness or shame.

Professor van der Kolk says that 'people with PTSD develop an enduring vigilance for and sensitivity to environmental threat' (van der Kolk 1997), leading to chronic elevation of the stress response. The accumulation of these stress hormones from trauma can have various negative effects on both our physical and mental wellbeing. Someone experiencing symptoms of PTSD may have some of the following symptoms, but not necessarily all of them:

- Intrusive memories

- Difficulty in staying present

- Flashbacks

- Emotional distress – easily and sometimes inappropriately triggered

- Hypervigilance and anxiety

- Avoidance of people, places and situations related to the trauma

- Nightmares and insomnia

- Easily startled

- Chronic fatigue

- Dissociation – not able to really engage in an experience or the feeling of not being in the body

- Difficulties in concentrating – brain fog

- Angry outbursts

- Memory lapses

- Irrational thoughts

- Chronic bouts of anxiety and/or depression.

WHY IT'S IMPORTANT TO ACKNOWLEDGE A HISTORY OF TRAUMA

To fully recover from an illness such as Long Covid, proper convalescence is needed together with periods of deep relaxation and rest. However, this is much more difficult for those who may be stuck in a fight, flight or freeze response for much of the time. The discomfort of acknowledging past trauma means it is common to be totally unaware of the impact of PTSD, since our culture encourages us to carry on, repress uncomfortable feelings and put on a brave face. This attitude (although perceived as normal because it's what most people do) is an impediment to recovery. Slowing down, resting and stopping, which is what chronic illness asks of us, means that we can no longer distract ourselves with 'doing' and being constantly on the go. Instead, we need to face our symptoms, including our emotions, as they arise. This can be very challenging.

For anyone with a history of chronic stress or PTSD, connecting to the body or breath in a yoga practice may initially be overwhelming. Being aware of the body and emotional sensations (also known as somatic experiencing or interoception) may, at first, induce uncomfortable reactions such as agitation, anxiety and distress. Although somatic/body awareness is part of what we are teaching in yoga therapy, this may trigger memories of past trauma. We therefore encourage you to go gently through the practices in this book, and to seek additional support from a trauma-informed therapist.

HOW DO OUR BODIES STORE EMOTIONS?

Emotions are not solely held in the brain. Imagine biting into a lemon. You may be pulling a face recalling the bitter, sour taste. By recognizing this, we can understand that emotions also involve physiological responses in the body. Traumatic experiences activate the stress response changing our heart rate, breathing, muscle tension and other bodily sensations. But these physical responses are intertwined with the emotional experience as well, creating a whole body connection. During a traumatic event, specific parts of the brain (including the premotor cortex, which helps us plan movement) encode emotional and physical responses. This can create an imprint of the trauma, linking specific movements, bodily sensations and emotions together. As a result, if triggered by reminders, individuals may experience similar emotional and physical reactions that are associated with the original traumatic event. These can show up as flashbacks, heightened anxiety, uncomfortable bodily sensations or a sense of being overwhelmed. For example, if someone is reminded of a trauma, their shoulders may tighten, they may hunch over their front body (an evolutionary mechanism to protect the organs when under threat) and their breathing will become shallow and rapid. This reaction is likely to be below the level of conscious awareness.

Understanding trauma and how it is held in the body is a complex and evolving field. Multiple brain regions are involved and research is still ongoing to fully comprehend the intricate connection between trauma, emotions and the body. What we do know is that yoga can markedly reduce symptoms of PTSD (van der Kolk 2015). In terms of yoga philosophy, it is considered that trauma affects specific *chakras*, depending on the type of experience. We explore how working with our *chakras* can help us to release stored tensions in Chapters 6 and 7.

LET'S PRACTISE: Cross body moving

Engaging in movements that replicate childhood patterns such as crawling can have multiple positive effects, including enhancing coordination, reducing impulsive behaviour and down-regulating hyperarousal of the nervous system (the stress response). Crossing the midline of our bodies facilitates communication between the brain's left and right hemispheres. This aids in brain reorganization such as resetting the motor cortex, and allows for balanced reliance on both hemispheres. Practising this is therefore very helpful for everyday activities such as walking and climbing stairs, as well as for higher cognitive skills such as reading and writing. This practice can also be done seated, or kneeling.

1. Begin by finding a position that is comfortable; if you are on your hands and knees, you might like to use a blanket under your knees. Ensure you feel balanced in your body by bringing hands under shoulders, knees under hips. Allow space between the hands and knees, space between the fingers, and visualize the length of your spine.

2. Take time to become aware of where your body is in the space around you. Sense the ground beneath you, and begin to observe the breath – just as it is.

3. There are two options to choose from, sitting or kneeling.

4. From sitting, place your hands on your knees. Lift up your right hand and, at the same time, your left foot as you inhale, then drop them down on the exhale. Repeat on the other side, lifting the left hand a few centimetres off the knee and lifting the right foot, then dropping them both down. Continue with this movement, lifting the opposite hand and foot, so you are marching on the spot from sitting. Practise five times on each side, then rest.

5. From kneeling on hands and knees, come into a Cat/tabletop position with the hands under the shoulders and knees under the hips. You are going to crawl to move forwards, using the opposite hand and knee. Take a hand's pace forward with your right hand and, at the same time, bring the left knee forward. Then take your left hand and your right knee forward. Continue with this crawling movement using opposite limbs, for as long as is comfortable, depending on your energy levels. Then rest.

6. If you wish, you could continue to practise, adding arm and leg extensions to this movement practice. Inhaling, lift and extend the left arm and right leg, lowering on the exhale. Inhaling, lift and extend the right arm and left leg, lowering on the exhale. This is quite dynamic, so pay attention to your energy levels and rest when you need to.

7. Repeat five times.

8. Slowly, gently, come down to the ground and rest for a few minutes before going back into your day.

KEEPING IT SIMPLE

The experience of trauma can have negative long-term cognitive effects affecting memory, attention, planning and problem solving – common experiences for those with chronic fatigue. For this reason, we advise you to take time to process the material in this chapter because this is key to understanding and increasing awareness of how your nervous system responds to particular situations. This will then help you to recognize which yoga tools to apply to support your recovery, not just on the mat, but in life, too. Recovery is like a jigsaw, and processing trauma may be a part of solving your puzzle.

CREATING A SAFE RESOURCE

Accessing a *Safe Resource* at times when we feel challenged allows us to be reminded of sensations of warmth, safety, comfort and peace, especially if anxiety, or panic, is triggered. A Safe Resource helps promote self-regulation and provides a refuge in difficult moments. It serves as a tool for grounding and self-soothing. Qualities we look for in a Safe Resource are often connected with memories of supportive people and places.

To develop a Safe Resource, think of a time, person, image or place when you felt happy, warm, joyful and supported. This image or place should hold connections to calm, positive memories or sensations. A Safe Resource may also be a real tactile object like a smooth stone, crystal or cloth, or perhaps a scent that brings peace and calm.

Examples of a Safe Resource

- Photo/image of a loved one, or a special place with comforting associated memories

- Smooth pebble

- Soft or silky cloth or item of clothing

- A scent, perhaps aromatherapy oil or scented candle

- Soft toy

- Item of jewellery

- Beads, crystals or stones

- Item or memory connected to a loved one such as a friend, teacher or relative who provides support

- Memory of a safe place – maybe in nature

- Image (real or imagined) of a loved pet

- Part of the body that feels safe, such as the softness of the palms.

For some, a Safe Resource will be to focus on the rhythm of the breath. For others this will trigger anxiety, which is why a Safe Resource is a very personal thing.

For the following practice we make suggestions such as using music or a pleasant scent to help calm the nervous system. Ultimately, in yoga we want to encourage a calm and peaceful mind as we work towards quieting the senses. This is one of the eight limbs described by Patanjali in the *Yoga Sutras*. However, for someone with trauma, being silent may be overwhelming, so soft music and safe smells may assist relaxation. Please note, we don't want to over-stimulate with sound or scents, especially with a client group who may have histamine issues (MCAS), so we need to use these tools carefully and be guided by the client.

LET'S PRACTISE: Developing a Safe Resource

1. Begin by choosing a space in which to practise that brings a sense of calm.

2. You may wish to play peaceful soothing music (please ensure it is low level because loud noise can impact the nervous system), or to have a soothing scent in the background, or photographs or pictures nearby that bring a sense of peace.

3. If feelings of sadness, fear, distress or anger arise during the session, use the safety of the space around you to direct your attention to sensory details. So, for example, you may look at the ceiling or the furniture to feel more present and held in your space.

4. Gaze at the floor or at your fingertips if the internal sensations you are noticing feel overwhelming. Be aware of your feet on the ground or the softness of your hands, and allow yourself to feel that you are as present as possible in the space that you are in.

5. Visualize your Safe Resource in as much detail as possible.

6. Allow yourself to see the specific colours, textures, sounds and scent that accompany this resource.

7. Give yourself permission to connect to positive emotions that connect with this resource.

8. If your Safe Resource is imagined, it may be a good idea to focus on something tangible such as a piece of cloth, a stone or crystal you can hold, or a photograph that can help to connect you to that imagined place, person or image.

9. Regular practice when you are resting or practising yoga allows you to more easily connect to your Safe Resource at times when you are encountering challenges or when you notice anxiety or feelings of disconnection.

THE SURVIVAL PERSONALITY

Many of those who experience chronic illness such as Long Covid previously had very busy, active lives, being the kind of people who find it hard to rest and be still. In some cases, they may have a form of high-functioning anxiety. These qualities are often normalized in Western culture and regarded as admirable. The ability to carry on regardless, to keep going through illness and pain, working harder and harder, ignoring the need for rest and self-regulation, is often applauded and seen as a strength rather than a liability. We can become so adept at this that we may feel uncomfortable if our stress levels drop, simply because we don't feel safe coming out of our busy heads. This is why resting, even to recover from illness, can be challenging when we are trapped in the cycle of constant doing. We just don't want to 'feel'.

The consistent repression and distraction from difficult emotions and the inability to relax, together with an extremely busy lifestyle, is often an indication of something known as the 'survival personality'. This may be a result of childhood trauma. Trauma expert Dr Gabor Maté describes the survival personality, also known as the type C personality, as someone able to suppress negative emotions such as anger, while maintaining a strong and happy facade.

Repression of emotions threaten not only our psychological health, but also our physical wellbeing by suppressing our immune system. This is because any kind of suppression, even if unconscious, causes stress to the CNS. So, for example, when asked how we are, we may say 'I'm fine, I'm really well/good/happy', when actually we are struggling to balance relationships, work and life in general. We may not even recognize our inability to express ourselves authentically because we have disconnected from our needs so effectively we don't know what it means to be our genuine, vulnerable self. This adds tension to our system, at an unconscious level. This type of repression can lead to a susceptibility to bacterial and viral invaders, or even to internal malignant changes. Type C personalities have also been correlated with chronic autoimmune and neurodegenerative conditions (Maté 2022).

Dr Maté (2022) describes certain characteristics of the survival personality. Perhaps some of these resonate with you – they certainly do with us:

- An automatic and compulsive concern for the emotional needs of others, alongside the ability to ignore one's own needs

- Identification with social roles, duty and responsibility

- Perfectionist qualities, overdriven and externally focused

- Often multi-tasking rather than doing one thing at a time

- A conviction that one must justify one's existence by doing and giving

- Repression of self-protective aggression and anger

- Harbouring beliefs such as 'I am responsible for how other people feel' and 'I must never disappoint anyone'. (Maté 2022, p.101)

Our emotional coping styles are shaped during childhood, and when we understand how emotions trigger our stress response, we can be more aware of how this contributes to illness. Chronic illness may appear to be primarily genetic, hence we see health conditions transmitted across generations in families. However, we can also understand how living with a dysregulated nervous system from an early age impacts our health and this may, of course, apply to whole family systems. *It is not just an outside agent like a pathogen that creates disease, but is also the 'territory'.* If we have had a history of stress and trauma, then we have the scenario set for reduced immunity and the likelihood of developing chronic disease. This is why it is inaccurate to label any illness as either 'physical' or 'psychological'. There is no such thing – we are holistic beings, something yoga also explains, with the mind and body being part of this.

BOUNDARIES, AND PEOPLE PLEASING

A survival personality also describes someone who struggles to establish boundaries, or has difficulty in saying 'no'. When we regularly prioritize others' needs over our own, we neglect self-care and move further away from our authentic self. You may have heard the term 'people pleaser'. However, this reduces what is, in effect, a survival mechanism to a personality trait. In reality, 'people pleasing' often originates from childhood as a need to be excessively and intuitively aware of other people's emotions in order to safeguard ourselves by staying attached to caregivers, or by being compliant. 'Fawning' is sometimes the phrase used when we think of this response, and is a behaviour that offers the illusion of soothing or keeping the nervous system calm in otherwise overwhelming circumstances. It is, in fact, an adaptive coping strategy, learned at a time when we may have been unable to process our emotions (for example, because of age) without the support of co-regulation. So, what we may think of as a 'personality flaw' is, in fact, an adaptive survival technique designed by our highly intelligent nervous systems to keep us safe. However, it can also be problematic because all too often we find ourselves in dysfunctional relationships and difficult circumstances, which undermines our ability to heal.

LET'S PRACTISE: Rocking to recover

1. For this practice, you need to be able to lie down on your back. Take a moment or two to become aware of your body and the way it meets the support beneath you. Allow yourself to let go – even if by one extra per cent. Pay particular attention to areas such as the jaw and shoulders, allowing them to soften. Observe how you are feeling now – mind, body and emotions. Allow everything to be as it is, bringing a sense of acceptance to however you are in this moment, even if difficult things are present such as pain or fatigue, tightness or difficulty in breathing. See if you can accept and even welcome these parts of you, feeling them just as sensations.

2. Roll onto your right side. Have the arms straight out in front of you at shoulder level, with the left palm resting on the right palm. Bend your knees slightly.

3. Start to stroke the left hand along the inner right arm, slowly drawing it up to the shoulder, then over the chest and finally opening the left arm wide to the left. As you do this you will roll onto your back. The lower part of the body is still in a slight twist. Take a few breaths in this position.

4. When you are ready, take the left hand and place it back gently on the chest, then stroke towards the right shoulder, then softly down the inner right arm and rest the hand back on top of the right palm. Rest and observe how you are from this movement. Repeat once or twice, moving slowly and mindfully as you stroke along the inner arm, rolling onto your back, then coming back onto your side.

5. Now cradle the side of the head with your right hand and bring the left hand in front of the belly. Using pressure with the left hand, begin to rock yourself by pressing down into the ground with the hand. Experiment with what feels most nourishing for you – rocking fast or slow. Take as much time as you need.

6. Now roll onto your back or front and rest, observing how you are.

7. When you are ready, roll onto your left side, arms in front at shoulder level, palms together, with the knees slightly bent. Taking your time, draw the right hand slowly along the inner left arm, across the shoulder and then the chest, finally opening the arm wide like a cross to the right side as you roll onto your back with the upper body. Pause for a few breaths, then return by taking the right hand to the chest and stroking slowly along the chest and down the arm until the palms come together. Repeat once or twice more.

8. As you did on the other side, rock yourself by cradling the side of the head in the left hand and by bringing the right hand in front of the belly. Pushing on the hand, softly rock yourself. Explore the rocking with curiosity.

9. Come back to your resting position and relax, focusing on your breath or Safe Resource.

HOW YOGA VIEWS TRAUMA

Yoga philosophy suggests that we are born with certain tendencies (*vasanas*) inherited from past lives and from our ancestors. We may then develop additional *vasanas* because of trauma in our current life. Our *vasanas* evolve into coping patterns (*samskaras*), such as those we saw described by the type C personality.

These patterns create something called a *kavacam* (like a veil or invisible mask), which is used to protect us from pain and difficult emotions. For example, we may become controlling, which gives us a sense of predictability, even though we never know what is going to happen next. Or we may develop a *kavacam* of being successful and busy or of being perfect, to keep us operating at a superficial level and to prevent those we encounter from getting too close. We see this on social media, where people post up idealized versions of themselves that don't actually reveal their true, vulnerable self. It's common for us to communicate from *kavacam* to *kavacam*, rather than from a place of authenticity. Having a *kavacam* in place is usually unconscious and is very exhausting because we are, in essence, working hard to keep up a false persona. Trauma, however, always has something to teach us about our patterns, our identities and our *kavacam* if we are willing to investigate and inquire within. Having a sense of faith and trust in life (*sraddha*) and letting go of control is one way we might slowly move forward, with the help of a trusted trauma-informed yoga therapist. As we heal from trauma, yoga considers that we are also healing for our ancestors by processing collective trauma. This happens as we explore emotional places that may have been suppressed for generations, allowing feelings and sensations to metabolize and release.

LET'S PRACTISE: Shaking it all out

It can be challenging to remain with our emotions. This next practice invites intentional shaking of hands and feet, and may feel energizing and refreshing, but do be aware of the need to rest afterwards (or during), and please bring a sense of gentleness to the shaking.

1. Begin by sitting in a chair or lying down. You could also stand for this practice if able. Become aware of your body in contact with the support and the feeling of your feet on the ground if you are sitting.

2. Notice the movement of the breath in and out of the nose (if this is comfortable, otherwise just focus on the movement of the belly).

3. Begin to gently wiggle the fingers and then the toes.

4. Allow the feet and hands to settle. Wiggle the fingers again and this time invite the movement of your hands, flapping, wiggling or gently circling the wrists. Soften the elbows. Encourage the movement to feel like a jiggle or a gentle shake.

5. Allow the shoulders to join this movement. Remember, it doesn't need to look like anything – we encourage curiosity of any sensation.

6. Slow the movement down and stop when you feel ready. Become aware of the breath again.

7. Wiggle the toes, lift the feet off the ground (you can do this one at a time, or both together). Let the movement continue upwards to the ankles, knees and across the hips, if that feels good.

8. Slow the movement down, then stop and bring your feet back to the ground. Just observe.

9. You can now move to shaking everything out, hands, feet, legs and arms, in a slow, rhythmic way. Remember, always move gently, with no forcing, encouraging a jiggle and shake rather than a jolt.

10. You may like to imagine shaking off whatever is on your mind at that moment. Imagine shaking it all off...

11. After a few moments come back to stillness. Become aware of your breath.

12. Notice how the body feels. What word comes to mind?

13. Rest for a few minutes or as long as is comfortable.

POLYVAGAL THEORY

In order to understand how yoga can help those with PTSD and Long Covid, it's useful to have an understanding of Polyvagal Theory (PVT). Trauma, particularly if severe or chronic, can dysregulate the vagus nerve. The vagus nerve is our longest cranial nerve and plays a crucial role in various important functions of the body. Often known as 'the wanderer' because it wanders about and stimulates the nerves through the entire length of the torso, the vagus nerve connects the brain and the gut and wraps itself around all the major organs. It is a key component of the PNS, which, as we saw previously, is responsible for promoting rest, relaxation and restoration. The vagus nerve is linked to many of the body systems, controlling functions such as heart rate, breathing, digestion and the immune response. Trauma-related vagal dysregulation can, however, lead to symptoms such as rapid heartbeat, shallow breathing, digestive problems and a suppression of the immune system.

PVT, developed by Dr Stephen Porges (2011), explains that there is a three-part hierarchical structure to our nervous system that reflects the way we react to the world around us. In understanding these, we can better support ourselves in our journey to recovery. Ultimately, PVT is about how we can feel safe and interact effectively with others in any circumstance. Again, yoga can play a key role here, which is why it's helpful to understand how PVT works.

The ventral vagal system

When our vagus nerve has optimal tone and is functioning effectively, the ventral vagal system (VVS) is online. Dr Porges calls this system the *social engagement system* as it enables social connection and safety by affecting our facial expressions, emotions and interactions with others. Being around supportive, compassionate people we trust activates this system, prompting closeness and better communication because of the sense of safety such a community provides. When we are in this autonomic state, we feel curious and open to possibility, and the world feels like a safe place.

The sympathetic nervous system

When we feel threatened, we initially rely on the VVS to resolve the situation, through social connection. This means that we may seek connection or support from others to feel secure again. However, if this doesn't work (maybe we don't have good social support or trusted friends, or maybe our family lives far away, for example), or because the threat is severe, our body switches to fight or flight. This describes the SNS that we saw in the previous chapter, in which stress hormones flood the body to help us to fight or run away from a situation that we perceive as threatening. When we are in this autonomic state, we may feel like running away, or that the world around us is threatening and harmful.

The dorsal vagal system

If fighting or running away doesn't resolve the situation, another part of the nervous system is immediately activated called the dorsal vagal system (DVS). Also related to the PNS, this older evolutionary response helps us to survive in life-threatening circumstances when there's no escape. It leads to immobilization and shutdown. We can see this in the wild when an animal may freeze if it is being chased, in order to protect itself by 'playing dead'. In other words, our DVS comes online under conditions of severe threat and we shut down. When we survive such a trauma, we may be left with symptoms such as dizziness, nausea or fatigue. Consequently, a common response, if we are triggered by something that unconsciously reminds us of such an event, is to disengage and dissociate from our body and surroundings. An example of how this may present in our thoughts is: 'I'm stuck, there's no point, I just don't care anymore.'

To use an example, those with Long Covid may have a great fear of reinfection, particularly if they were breathless, hospitalized or ventilated. This fear can trigger a memory of the original illness, and so the reaction may be to become hypervigilant (SNS) or to freeze (DVS) if they encounter situations where there could be Covid. Examples of these could be in crowds of unmasked people, on an aeroplane, or if news of new variants is spotlighted by the media. We may see the last two of these states (SNS or DVS) in a yoga class. For example, someone may present as being very detached and disengaged or, conversely, highly anxious.

WORKING WITH THE BODY AND TRAUMA

From reading this chapter, we can understand that the body holds on to traumatic events (van der Kolk 2015). Therefore, it is necessary to connect to the body slowly and kindly so that we can mindfully develop a relationship with our sensations. To begin with, we focus on the here-and-now in a way that helps us to feel more grounded and resourced. It's important to note that even focusing on safety has to be offered as a choice. It cannot be forced, and nor do we want to override any felt experience of distress, defensiveness or tension. What we seek is a safe-enough space that allows us to notice and ultimately be with our reactions. Creating a Safe Resource, together with a safe space in which to practise and a safe connection with a trusted therapist, are essential parts of allowing this process to begin. Please note that exploring interoceptive skills by going inwards may be initially challenging and even distressing. Because bodily sensations may be overwhelming and uncomfortable, we recommend working with a trauma-informed yoga therapist or mental health professional to gain a sense of safety slowly, over time. An experienced therapist works using titration, which means coming in and out of bodily sensations as appropriate. We don't cover this here because this is something that needs an individual approach.

LET'S PRACTISE: Soothing sounds

Research suggests that certain sounds are one of the most powerful ways to tone the vagus nerve, together with slow breathing, which we cover in more detail in the next chapter. In yoga, Vedic chanting and sounding using *mantra* is a central part of many traditions. For the following practice we invite you to use either the chant 'Om', or the humming breath, which we introduced in Chapter 1, when we hummed on the exhalation.

Om

Om is a sacred sound, said to have been made as the universe was created, and also said to incorporate all sounds. It is a very powerful mantra and helps the movement of *prana* (energy). In terms of science, certain sounds have been shown to tone the vagus nerve, leading to VVS, which is what we want. 'Om' is often mispronounced – the sound to aim for is 'Om', as in 'home'.

Let's practise: Om

1. Come to a comfortable sitting position.

2. If you can, have your head, neck and spine in line, and take a moment or two to observe the space between the crown of the head and the tailbone.

3. Inhale.

4. As you exhale, bring your mouth into a circle and from the belly make the sound 'ooooo'; as the breath begins to fade, bring the lips slowly together so the end of the breath sounds 'mmm'.

5. Chant 3–5 times on the exhale.

6. If you are not comfortable with this mantra, you may like to hum the breath out instead.

POLYVAGAL THEORY AND THE *GUNAS*: A NOTE FOR TEACHERS AND THERAPISTS

From a yogic perspective, PVT relates to the *gunas*. For example, the ventral vagal tone describes a *sattvic* response when we are in a state of flow and connection. The SNS of activation relates to the state of *rajas*. The dorsal vagal tone describes the heavier, sleepier *guna* of *tamas*. We need a healthy balance of these three *gunas* when appropriate. For example, we need a little of the SNS (*rajas*) to get going and to be motivated when we are working or have a task to complete. The dorsal vagal tone (*tamas*) is helpful if we need to sleep or deeply relax. Ultimately, we want to be in ventral vagal tone (*sattva*) for much of the time, so that we are happy, clear and in the flow. Understanding where we are with these three states of being – whether we are using the *guna* model or PVT – is very helpful for our healing.

LET'S PRACTISE: Somatic grounding

Soma means body in Latin, so somatic means of the body. In this practice we aim to connect to the body, sensing our surroundings and support (like the floor, chair, bed or mat). This engenders a feeling of security as we remind ourselves that we are always held by the Earth.

1. Find a comfortable place to lie down, or to sit.

2. Feel your feet on the ground if you are sitting. If you are lying, notice how your body feels in contact with your support. Bring attention to all the parts of the body that meet the support. Visualize yourself relaxing and being held.

3. If you are sitting, allow your feet to explore the surface beneath you, so that you feel fully in contact with the floor.

4. If you are lying, take time to get comfortable. Wriggle, roll from side to side and feel the way that your body senses the floor, or support. If comfortable to do so, close your eyes, but notice if this feels challenging. If so, soften your gaze and allow your eyes to remain open.

5. Begin to tune into your breath. If following your breath makes you anxious, just stay with the sensation of being in contact with your support. If anything feels too much, use your Safe Resource to bring a sense of calm.

6. Placing a hand on the belly, begin to sense the breath.

7. Follow the gentle rise and fall of the belly with each breath under your hand.

8. Inhaling, repeat, either out loud or silently, 'Inhaling compassion'.

9. Exhaling, repeat, either out loud or silently, 'Exhaling peace'.

10. If you prefer not to follow your breath at this time, continue to focus on the feeling of the parts of your body in contact with your support.

11. If you find your mind is jumping around, just notice this. Without judgement, come gently back to the breath or the feeling of your body/feet in contact with the ground or your support. Observe the natural spaces between the thoughts.

12. Repeat this process of noticing thoughts and coming back to the breath or the sensation and feeling of your feet/body and its relationship to the surface you are lying or sitting on, for as long as is comfortable to you. Use your Safe Resource at any time you need to.

13. There is nothing to do, nowhere to go, no particular way to breathe, so just let yourself be here at this moment, noticing thoughts without judgement.

14. Observe if you feel the need to move, and allow yourself to feel this as a sensation for a moment before moving.

15. Begin to wriggle your fingers and toes.

16. Move slowly and gently in ways that feel comforting.

17. If you are lying, perhaps hug the knees into the chest, rocking out from side to side, or stretching out your arms.

18. Take all the time you need before you come back to your daily life.

THE WINDOW OF TOLERANCE

For those experiencing PTSD, it is not unusual for our nervous system to switch from the states of extreme anxiety to a freeze, shutdown state. What we are aiming for in a yoga practice is to widen this window, so that we become more present, more in the flow of life, more rested and replenished. In other words, yoga can move us towards a state of ventral vagal tone (*sattva*) and away from the extreme swings of anxiety and dissociation. The good news is that although we know our body stores traumatic memories, it also holds the key to recovery. Engaging our social nervous system (ventral vagal tone) is therefore a crucial part of healing.

We can promote good vagal tone using specific practices which encourage awareness of each of the vagal states. Some yoga tools promote soothing and calm (ventral vagal tone), some are more mobilizing and activating (SNS) and some promote inner stillness and deep rest (dorsal vagal tone). We give examples of these in later chapters. In each case, awareness of how we are by monitoring our body sensations and understanding how the nervous system is responding is key, because it encourages and empowers us to practise in a way that can change our state when needed.

NADYNE'S STORY

I've always been a plate spinner. In fact, it was something I prided myself on. I worked in the City for many years and was up at 5am to get to the gym, followed by a full day at work, followed by more exercise and then out with colleagues or clients. This was my pattern, and taking on more and more plates to spin was something I celebrated. I loved to exercise. Hard. When I left the City I retrained as a personal trainer, then a yoga therapist and then a psychotherapist. But it was only when I got Covid I realized that I was not able to do all the things I had loved to do.

When I got ill, it was during a very stressful time in my life. I was taking exams for my yoga therapy qualification and in the middle of a divorce. I was surprised to find my symptoms were a lot worse than I expected. But, even in the acute stage, I didn't really stop, despite feeling exhausted and unwell. I was well practised at overriding my feelings to keep going.

Having Covid was my first experience of breathlessness, and the sheer panic I felt at not being able to breathe was scary. I became quite fearful about many things at that time. Even when I recovered, I was frightened to venture back outside, although the government guidelines said I could. But I really wanted to get back to normal! Eventually, I went for a short walk and was shocked to discover how fatigued I felt, after such a small amount of activity. This was my introduction to the many symptoms of Long Covid.

I felt very lonely during this long period of illness, which reminded me of my teen years when I had been diagnosed with post-viral fatigue. That was also an incredibly isolating and scary time. Consequently, I tried to get back into my normal activities pretty much straight away, but found that I couldn't. My wellbeing has always been very much based on physical exercise and dynamic yoga. I can see now that these patterns of constant doing, achieving and keeping active were an adaptation to my early childhood, which was often chaotic. My father was a heavy drinker who sadly died in a car accident when I was only 12. This was very traumatic. In my grief, I poured myself into schoolwork. In later years this turned into studying hard, working hard, exercising hard, partying hard...pretty much anything other than facing how I was really feeling.

It was only when I developed Long Covid that I slowly realized the power of radical rest. Our society talks about rest as if it's a nice idea, but my previous life didn't allow for that, what with work and family and studying, and my need to exercise. Eventually, my body said no, and I was forced to stop. And yes, it was hard. I felt like a rebel when I was resting because it seemed so unfamiliar! It was the ultimate challenge to face myself in this way, knowing that the distractions I had used to stay away from my feelings were no longer available, and my emotional inner world, which had been buried for years, had to be finally acknowledged and accepted. I've learned now to view this time of chronic illness with a deep sense of compassion.

It took time to properly recover and heal because, as a plate spinner, I set myself up for continual relapse and debilitating fatigue for many months by overdoing things before I was ready. I eventually realized I needed to reframe my life and I took a step back from the activities I had used to cope with stress. So many of my clients tell me they have no idea how they managed to do what they did before they had this condition. I was the same. But Long Covid taught me some transformative lessons.

I'm grateful for learning to rest, to breathe better, to take time for myself when I need to – without waiting for my body to crash. I still have times when I relapse – I'm only human after all – and my perfectionist patterns trick me into thinking I can still do everything. But having Long Covid taught me that my body is wise, and if I listen to it, and don't ignore the whispers, I can live the life I want to live. And it's a better life.

TRAUMA-INFORMED TIPS FOR THERAPISTS

- *Encourage curiosity.* Invite students to move in ways that feel good for them and not simply by following your directions. By allowing the student the agency to practise as they wish and staying within their window of tolerance, students can become curious about when, why and how they meet their boundaries (i.e., when they need to stop and rest), without feeling that they 'should' be doing exactly what they are told to do. This might look like noticing sensations of their body in contact with the floor, or how different ways of moving affect their breath and their emotional state. In this way, they are learning not to push against cues of fatigue, breathlessness or pain, and are learning to pace.

- *Encourage personal choice.* Everything must always be a *choice* – we are aiming to give the student back their agency. The practice of deciding whether to participate in something is incredibly powerful. Those with trauma feel excessively disempowered, so we need to teach in a way where our language is not about instruction but is always offering choice. The use of invitational language is key (and we gave guidance on wording in the last chapter), as is stressing the importance of feeling free to ignore anything that doesn't feel beneficial. By inviting people to listen to their inner voice, and to be guided by the breath (if appropriate) and by what feels good, we empower the student. This personal agency within the practice, with time, will transfer into many aspects of life. For example, we might invite our students to follow the breath, but always with the option of focusing on their Safe Resource, if following the breath makes them too anxious.

- *We advise no hands on assists or adjustments.* There is no need to place anyone's body into a shape it doesn't feel comfortable to be in. As teachers, we do not know what is best for the student. They are experts in themselves. Touch should be invitational and always with consent, if at all.

- *Eyes do not have to be closed.* For many trauma sufferers, removing sense of sight causes fear and hypervigilance, the very things we are aiming to avoid.

- *A heightened state of anxiety makes stillness and meditation challenging for some.* Invite permission to *not* do anything that feels uncomfortable, with no need for the student to give a reason.

A big part of recovery from trauma is relearning to breathe. This has a transformative impact on our nervous system, and is so important that the next three chapters explain how to breathe for wellness and energy. However, we know that for many who have Long Covid, working with the breath may induce feelings of anxiety and panic because it can trigger a reminder of times when it was difficult to breathe. Please know that we honour and respect this, and that learning to rebreathe is something to be done gently and slowly when the time is right. This also applies to healing from trauma. Understandably, we may wish to rush through the practices in order to heal faster. However, it's important to recognize and acknowledge that time and space are essential to allow the journey towards recovery to unfold. We explore in later chapters how acceptance of the present moment, learning to listen to our bodies and cultivating self-compassion will help us on this journey.

KEY POINTS

- ✓ Trauma is subjective and describes any experience that disrupts and overwhelms our ability to cope.

- ✓ Trauma can occur when there is not enough time, space or support to heal and recover from stress.

- ✓ Experiencing trauma in childhood affects how our body responds to stress later in life, and can make us more susceptible to chronic illness (due to dysregulation of the nervous system).

- ✓ PTSD and C-PTSD symptoms can make it more difficult to recover from illness due to the discomfort of 'resting' and stillness.

- ✓ Our body stores emotional responses, and memories of trauma can be triggered unconsciously via physical movement, breath awareness and certain circumstances that may remind us of the original trauma. This is why we always go gently when working with those with a history of trauma.

- ✓ We recommend working with a trauma-informed therapist to guide and support recovery if you have trauma symptoms.

- ✓ Creating a Safe Resource can assist cultivation of calm and grounding. It is very important to practice in a safe place with a trusted 'other' such as a trained trauma-informed therapist.

- ✓ Many survivors of trauma learn to repress and distract from difficult emotions, by staying busy and ignoring their emotional needs. Dr Gabor Maté defines this as the 'survival personality'.

- ✓ Polyvagal Theory (PVT), developed by Dr Stephen Porges, assists in our understanding of how we can learn to feel safe in our bodies as we become more aware of the three different states of the nervous system.

- ✓ Yoga must be offered as a trauma-informed practice where everything is invitational and a choice.

- ✓ Yoga can empower individuals who have experienced trauma by offering them the opportunity to become curious, move in ways that feel good and to encounter safe levels of challenge.

Chapter 3

BREATHING FOR WELLBEING: ACCESSING THE NERVOUS SYSTEM

Eastern traditions like yoga have long understood the power of the breath. In Chapter 5 we explore how *prana*, or life force energy, can be harnessed by breathing consciously to assist recovery. However, it's important to note that modern science is also now adding to the story, and research extolling the virtues of healthy breathing continues to uncover the vast benefits of learning to breathe well. This is great news for those with chronic health problems including Long Covid, because it offers a very positive way forward. The next two chapters focus on functional breathing for wellbeing. We look at the restorative nature of the breath and how, by relearning to breathe, we can assist our body's ability to recover, restore and replenish.

BREATHING AND LONG COVID

There are many breathing issues associated with Long Covid. Even if you had mild Covid, you may have found yourself experiencing difficulties such as breathlessness that continued for many weeks after the initial illness had passed. In some cases, this may have been severe and hasn't yet been resolved. If you've ever suffered from breathlessness, you'll know how scary that feeling is. When our brain recognizes changes to our breathing rhythm, it responds immediately, alerting our nervous system to trigger the stress response. This is why the symptoms of dysfunctional breathing are often linked to feelings of anxiety and increased stress. It's not in your head!

Shortness of breath and gasping are common symptoms of the post-Covid picture, all of which impact daily life. You might find yourself getting out of breath when you walk up and down stairs, or perhaps you find yourself breathless when walking and talking. You might feel tight in the chest or notice that your breath quickens and your heart rate rises, even when you are resting. This type of breathing is known as a Breathing Pattern Disorder (BPD).

WHAT IS A BREATHING PATTERN DISORDER?

A BPD indicates a breathing rate in excess of our metabolic needs. There can be many causes, such as nervous system dysregulation (of which anxiety and chronic stress are often part of the picture), a medical condition, hormone fluctuations, biomechanics (movement and posture) and excessive heat, altitude, diet or anything that prevents normal respiration.

Unfortunately, BPDs remain widely under-diagnosed and under-treated, yet often contribute to ill health. A Long-Covid cardiopulmonary study conducted by Professor Donna Mancini MD, of the School of Medicine at Mount Sinai Hospital, found that several abnormalities, including reduced exercise capacity and abnormal breathing patterns that impacted daily life, were present in 88 per cent of participants with Long Covid (Mancini *et al.* 2021). Paradoxical breathing, also known as reverse breathing, in which the chest wall draws in on the inhalation and out on the exhalation, was also present, indicating a system under extreme stress. The study also found evidence of reduced blood flow to small blood vessels in the lungs, potentially due to micro blood clots, which we now know is also a part of the Long Covid set of symptoms for some people: 'These findings suggest that in a subgroup of long haulers, hyperventilation and/or dysfunctional breathing may underlie their symptoms. This is important as these abnormalities may be addressed with breathing exercises or "retraining"' (Mancini *et al.* 2021).

We urge anyone experiencing respiratory difficulties to see their GP or health professional before embarking on any breathing exercises. However, there are some small changes that you can make that will lead to big improvements in how you feel. Even if you are not aware of breathing difficulties, if you have symptoms of Long Covid or chronic fatigue or indeed any chronic illness, then please read on, as it is probable that dysfunctional breathing plays a part in your story.

WHY FUNCTIONAL BREATHING?

Many people, irrespective of Long Covid, go about their lives breathing in a way that isn't conducive for wellbeing or energy. We breathe approximately 20,000 times each day and yet, for many of us, these breaths go largely unnoticed. That is until we experience difficulties. These include any disturbances such as over-breathing, unexplained breathlessness or irregularity in breathing patterns.

WHAT IS DYSFUNCTIONAL BREATHING?

- Mouth breathing
- Movement from mainly the upper chest
- Audible breathing
- Frequent sighing

- Frequent yawning

- Paradoxical breathing (when the belly moves in on the inhale and out on the exhale)

- Breathing too fast.

Breathing dysfunctionally usually involves taking short rapid breaths often via the mouth, breathing from the chest and under-utilizing the diaphragm. This leads to chronic over-breathing, also known as hyperventilation. All these factors profoundly impact our health.

Oxygen is the gas that fuels energy production in the body, and as fatigue, PEM and circulatory issues are predominant symptoms of Long Covid, addressing the efficient uptake of oxygen and gas exchange is a key factor for recovery. Functional breathing places an emphasis on breathing slowly, smoothly and lightly in order to gently, but optimally, impact the whole system. The foundation to functional breathing is nasal breathing, which encourages the effective use of the diaphragm. We will explore this further in the next chapter.

Individuals experiencing chronic pain, anxiety or illness often breathe far more than average. Unless we bring conscious awareness to the breath, it is unlikely that we will notice how we actually breathe. However, each time we take a breath, we have the opportunity to become more aware so that we can change how we feel just by changing how we breathe.

LET'S PRACTISE: Breath awareness

1. Sit comfortably, or lie down on your back or on your front.

2. Notice how you feel, right now, without judgement. Let whatever comes into your mind be there. Just observe.

3. Take some time to focus on your breath.

4. If you can, focus on your next inhale.

5. Observe, without judgement, where the breath goes.

6. What parts of your body are moving as you breathe?

7. You may find it helpful to place a hand on the belly and a hand on your chest.

8. Notice any movement in these places. Perhaps you can feel a rise and fall of your chest or belly against your hand?

9. Begin to follow the journey of the breath as it moves in the body.

10. With each breath, just notice these movements as you inhale and exhale.

11. After a few minutes return to normal breathing, release your hand and observe how you feel.

12. Has anything changed? Take time to notice if you feel differently: physically, emotionally or mentally. Perhaps there are no changes. Know that learning to be more aware takes time, and that each day offers us a new opportunity to observe with curiosity and non-judgement.

Congratulations – you've spent some time meditating on the breath! Our breath gives us several thousand opportunities to meditate throughout the day simply by bringing our awareness to each inhalation and exhalation. Even by focusing on your breath for a few minutes, you will begin to see positive changes.

Experiencing any of the following symptoms may be a sign that you are not breathing functionally:

- Shortness of breath
- Insomnia
- Asthma, COPD (Chronic Obstructive Pulmonary Disease)
- Chronic cough
- Sinusitis and allergies
- Postural issues
- Heartburn
- Migraines
- Muscle cramps and muscle pain
- Exercise intolerance/PEM
- Poor memory and/or 'brain fog'
- High/low blood pressure
- Constipation
- Abdominal pain and/or IBS
- Lethargy
- Chronic fatigue

- Dizziness

- Cold hands and feet/Raynaud's syndrome

- Recurrent infections

- Anxiety and panic attacks

- Heart rate irregularities (please see a medical professional if this is the case).

If we were to put together a list of the symptoms being experienced under the umbrella term of 'Long Covid', we would see many, if not all, of these symptoms. We may spend much of our lives seeking treatment, and still find them unresolved. Perhaps you have had a number of highly sophisticated tests, only to be told that there is 'nothing identifiably wrong'. Perhaps you've even been told 'it's all in your head' or that you are anxious, experiencing hormonal/menopausal symptoms, or that you are even a hypochondriac. *The likelihood is that, unknowingly, what's not been addressed is how you are breathing. Yet healthy breathing is the very foundation of our wellbeing.*

In Chapter 1 we explored the impact of stress on the mind and body and how, by becoming more aware of the breath, we can communicate calm and safety to our nervous system. Although we recognize that other factors contribute to the Long Covid experience, in addressing BPDs, we give ourselves a better chance to manage stress, find balance, improve symptoms and encourage recovery.

A creative and playful way to help us become more aware of our breathing is to visibly 'draw' the breath. In his book *Draw Breath* Tom Granger advises us that actually 'drawing the breath' can bring attention to our breathing rhythm (Granger 2019).

LET'S PRACTISE: Drawing the breath

Take a piece of paper and a pencil. We are going to ride the wave of the breath and note it down.

1. Close your eyes and let the tip of the pencil find the paper.

2. Focus on your breath, and without any need to change anything, allow the pencil to move upwards as you inhale and downwards as you exhale.

3. Each wave that you draw represents a full breath.

4. It is unlikely that every breath is equal; some exhalations may be longer and some waves may appear smaller or larger on the paper.

5. Taking this time out to focus on the breath in this way allows us to bring awareness to our breathing rhythm.

Drawing the breath is a great mindfulness practice to help us observe our breathing rhythm. We can often see, by observing the breath in this way, that our breathing pattern is irregular. Our breath is unlikely to be a perfect wave. The inhale may not be equal to the exhale. The less perfect the curves of breath appear, the more likely it is that you are accurately drawing how you are actually breathing.

BREATHING TO REGULATE A DYSREGULATED NERVOUS SYSTEM

Our ANS is intricately linked to our breath. To move towards a more functional pattern, we want to practise breathing exercises that help to communicate to the brain that we are safe. By repeatedly stimulating the vagus nerve during slow breathing practices, we can shift the nervous system towards a more restful state, resulting in positive changes such as lower blood pressure, a lower heart rate and a general improved sense of wellbeing and calm.

Learning to breathe well is especially important for those experiencing dysautonomia, a disorder of the nervous system that is responsible for involuntary, automatic functions in the body. This means that we are, for the most part, unaware of our breathing, heart rate fluctuations and blood pressure changes. Dysautonomia may involve failure of the SNS and PNS parts of the ANS, and this can affect our pulse, digestion, bladder and sexual function and also our body/skin temperature. When these autonomic functions become erratic, our ability to regulate and restore balance to our system diminishes. Therefore, being able to regulate the nervous system via conscious awareness of the breath is vital.

LET'S PRACTISE: Taking a micro-breathing break

Making small changes on a daily basis is the most effective way to adopt new behaviours to assist recovery. It's important that we practise breathing when we are at rest, so that in the event that we notice challenges/stress, we are able to turn to our toolbox of well-practised breathing techniques. In the following practice, we explore how to take a minute out of the day, whatever we may be doing, to become more aware of our breathing. You might like to set a timer reminder on your phone to do this every few hours.

1. From either sitting or lying, just take a pause from whatever you are doing.

2. Feel the support of whatever it is that you are sitting or lying on.

3. Place one hand on the belly and the other on the chest.

4. Notice the breath, without the need to make any changes.

5. Begin to slow down the rhythm of the breath, feeling the movement of your hands on your body. This should be a comfortable rhythm. If you are gasping or forcing the breath in any way, return to your normal pattern.

6. Breathe in this way for about a minute – set a timer if you need to. If a minute is too long, make it slightly shorter.

IMPORTANT: GENTLE IS THE WAY

Because many people with Long Covid experience chronic fatigue, we need to be considerate with breathing practices so as not to over-tax the nervous system. Indeed, some breathing exercises can exacerbate symptoms, as we explained in the Guidance section in the Introduction.

Learning to breathe well takes time. Many people may have unknowingly been breathing dysfunctionally for years. We urge everyone to practise gently and with kindness when exploring the breath. Changes can take time, and that is okay. Being gentle with ourselves can be challenging for many reasons, and so our advice is to explore slowly, with curiosity and compassion. Never force the breath, and stop the exercise if you are uncomfortable. Remember, we are taking small steps here. If you find following the breath difficult, observe the movements of the body instead, and remember your Safe Resource is there for you if you need it.

WHAT KIND OF BREATHING IS BEST?

For a moment, let's think about how our breath affects our emotional state. The connection between the two is reciprocal – changes in one lead to changes in another. In other words, whenever we feel an emotion such as fear, excitement, happiness or anger, our breathing acts like a barometer for this. For example, if we are stressed, our breathing rate gets faster and becomes more shallow, and if we are calm and happy, the rate slows down. When we are calm, we feel stronger, we are better able to manage our symptoms and function from a more balanced place, because we are breathing more functionally.

LET'S PRACTISE: When life gives you lemons

We used the example of biting into a lemon in the previous chapter to explain how emotions are stored in the body. Here, using lemons again, we show how an experience also affects how we breathe.

1. Sit for a moment and make fists with your hands.

2. Squeeze them as tightly as you can.

3. Imagine you are squeezing two lemons to get as much juice from them as possible.

4. Did you notice what happens to your breath and face when you tighten and tense your muscles?

As well as breathing too fast, many of us hold our breath when we experience tension or are concentrating, such as in this practice. In order to change our breathing habits, we need to explore how we breathe when we are relaxing. If we can extend the exhalation, for example, we engage the PNS – the 'rest and digest' part of the nervous system. This calms us down if we are feeling stressed. The following exercise demonstrates this.

LET'S PRACTICE: Flower breathing

1. Sit comfortably and feel your feet on the ground, your back supported by the chair. We are going to start by moving our fingers in time with the breath, so take a moment or two to become aware of the difference between your inhalation and exhalation. Become conscious of your hands.

2. Place your hands on your lap, making a gentle fist with each hand, curling the fingers softly towards the palms of the hands.

3. As you inhale, uncurl the fingers, softly opening the palms like flowers slowly blooming to stretch out the fingers like petals. Exhale slowly and bring the fingertips gently together like buds, in time with a long, smooth out-breath if possible. If you can, extend the exhalation a little, so it's longer than your inhalation.

4. Imagine the petals furling and unfurling more slowly each time you breathe, opening on the in-breath and slowly folding in on the exhale. Practise for up to 10 breaths.

TECH (OR SCREEN) APNEA: HOW BEING ON SCREEN IMPACTS BREATHING

Tech (or screen) apnea is a new term used to describe the effects of technology on our breathing patterns. Regardless of stress levels, spending long periods of time on any screen, including scrolling on the phone, means that we are continuously distracted. We can become so absorbed in social media or our emails that we actually hold our breath as we forget to breathe enough. The term 'apnea' refers to under-breathing, where the breath becomes very shallow. This means we are mainly breathing into the chest and not breathing low enough to activate the diaphragm. This is an issue because holding our breath or breathing in this way is a signal of threat to the body and puts our system into a fight or flight response mode. According to Dr Stephen Porges (quoted in Gupta 2023), screen apnea is a manifestation of our body's stress response, and when we are faced with overwhelming stimuli, such as constant scrolling or never-ending emails, our nervous system looks for signals to decipher whether or not it's under threat. This begins a series of physiological changes including shallow breathing and slower heart rate to divert resources to help us to maintain focus. The more unexpected a stimuli is (such as receiving notification alerts), the more likely the body is to perceive that there is a threat. In other words, when notifications and alerts are constant, as is often the case, it shifts the nervous system into a state of dysregulation. Lack of movement from sitting in front of a screen also adds to the problem of screen apnea, as poor posture increases the effects of shallow breathing.

So how do we combat tech apnea? We practise conscious awareness of the breath and take regular time out to breathe properly, to move and stretch, away from screens. We suggest taking micro-breathing breaks during any time spent on screen (please see the practice 'Taking a micro-breathing break'). Our advice when recovering from Long Covid is to limit screen time as much as possible, because this is another source of over-stimulation that leads to fatigue, impacting negatively on our nervous system.

LET'S PRACTISE: Breath guiding movement, movement guiding breath – slowing down

This next practice allows us to connect the rhythm of our breath to gentle movement.

1. Either sit comfortably, or lie down with knees bent and arms by your sides.

2. Take time to feel the support beneath you.

3. As you take your next in-breath, if you are sitting, let the arms rise up by your sides, so they are level with the shoulders. If you are lying down, run your arms along the floor up and out beside you, to make snow angel shapes.

4. As you exhale, let the arms float back down to your sides, palms on your knees if you are sitting, or beside your hips if you are lying down.

5. Be guided by your breathing rhythm. Be curious about following the inhale and the exhale, with no need to move too far or to change anything.

6. Continue inhaling to raise the arms and exhaling to float the arms back down by the sides.

7. Now imagine that the air takes on a slightly thicker quality. Perhaps you are on the beach with your fingers trailing through the soft sand, or maybe you are gently floating through the warm waters of a tropical ocean. You choose.

8. Feel how this imagined quality of air begins to slow down the movement of the arms, and see how this guides the inhalation to become a little slower and the exhalation a little longer.

9. Take time to explore this idea. Remember, there is no rush to achieve anything. Breathing practices are a process to investigate, not a goal to achieve.

10. Take 5–10 of these slower breaths, using your breath to guide the movement. If at any time you feel tired or the movement is too much, stop. Only do as many as feels right.

11. Feel the ground or support beneath you and come back into the day.

THE CARBON DIOXIDE (CO2) STORY

We may think of CO_2 simply as a waste gas. However, when we consider breathing and our health, we need to look at CO_2 as well as oxygen (O_2). CO_2 has four essential roles:

- On the in-breath, CO_2 signals to the brainstem (via the phrenic nerve that tells the diaphragm to move downwards) to start an inhalation by lowering the pH level. This triggers breathing.

- CO_2 makes the smooth muscles of the airways relax so that they open and let air into the lungs.

- CO_2 also relaxes the smooth muscles in the blood vessels so that they dilate and increase circulation.

- Because CO_2 lowers the pH, this allows for greater release of oxygen from the blood into the cells.

In summary, CO_2 paves the way for better oxygen uptake to the cells. This means more energy and improved health and wellbeing.

WHAT DOES IT MEAN TO HYPERVENTILATE?

When we are stressed or anxious we hyperventilate, which means that we are breathing too fast. Consequently, we breathe off too much CO_2. This, in turn, keeps us in the stress response. Reduced levels of CO_2 cause blood vessels to constrict and may lead to a condition known as respiratory alkalosis, characterized by an increase in blood pH levels. This consequently restricts the flow of blood, impacting the delivery of oxygen to the body and brain. People prone to hyperventilation may actually experience as much as a 25 per cent reduction in fuel to the brain due to an imbalance of CO_2 and O_2. This lack of blood flow is very inefficient for focus, memory and clear thinking, and may contribute to the feeling of brain fog and tiredness that frequently accompanies Long Covid and fatigue states. As we know, stress increases hyperventilation, but this also incites anxiety, depression and fear, leading to further over-breathing and increased symptoms. We then end up in a cycle of breathing too fast, which further exacerbates stress, thus increasing fatigue and brain fog and delaying recovery.

When we have healthy amounts of CO_2 in the body, oxygen is delivered more effectively to the mitochondria, which are implicated in all kinds of functions including energy production. If we are exhaling too much CO_2, however, the effects can be quite drastic, including feelings of dizziness, lightheadedness, anxiety, panic and the other symptoms listed earlier. This is why slowing the breath down and breathing through the nose (discussed in the next chapter) can have such a positive impact on our health, as the correct exchange of gases will, in time, dramatically improve our health.

TO HOLD THE BREATH OR NOT?

The effect of low levels of CO_2 is also thought to have a direct impact on many conditions such as asthma and high blood pressure. Therefore, it's important to not only address oxygen levels but also to acknowledge that low levels of CO_2 in the blood compromise our health. The ability to take small pauses after the exhalation as we breathe demonstrates our ability to tolerate higher levels of CO_2. Many people refer to this as breath holding; however, we prefer to refer to it as a 'comfortable pause' (Rothenberg 2019). Our advice for people with Long Covid is that longer breath holds are *not* where we should begin for breath retraining as this will, in fact, overly tax the nervous and cardiovascular systems. Remember, we are trying to take the work out of breathing by inviting a gentle, slow breath.

Patrick McKeown, of The Oxygen Advantage® and Buteyko Method,[1] suggests that small breath holds after the exhalation, which he refers to as the 'control pause', can be a useful way of assessing body oxygen levels. The inability to comfortably maintain a pause after the exhale may indicate low CO_2 and alerts the respiratory system to breathe faster, creating the hallmark of chronic hyperventilation.

LET'S PRACTISE: The comfortable pause

This next practice demonstrates how you can monitor your comfort level of pausing after the exhalation. We would prefer you not to use a stopwatch, or to become fixated on holding the breath for a certain length of time. Instead, just observe the natural pause after the exhale, and become curious about the sensations arising as you slowly and gradually over time lengthen the pause, as you become more comfortable to do so. Please note that this practice advises you to breathe through the nose. There is more on this in the next chapter, but if you can't yet do this, skip this practice for now, and come back to it when you are ready.

1. Sitting comfortably, feel your feet on the floor and notice the sensation of support beneath you. You may wish to close your eyes. Take some time to come into your body, feeling yourself here. Take a gentle inhale through the nose. Exhale. Repeat two or three times.

---

1   https://buteykoclinic.com

2. Inhale gently through the nose. Exhale lightly.

3. Pause for a comfortable period of time. There should be no strain or forcing to hold the breath.

4. *Inhale as soon as you feel the need to breathe.* For many, this will be a very short period of time indeed.

5. Continue to breathe gently until you feel ready to explore the comfortable pause again.

> Breath holding, particularly for individuals prone to panic disorder or anxiety, may incite a strong fear response as past memories of breathing difficulties can be triggered. It is therefore essential that we practise gently and with compassion for our current state of health. We advise focusing on making very small changes that encourage functional breathing and going at your own pace. You may therefore wish to hold the breath for no more than a second or two after the exhale, or to not do this practice at all.

THE CELL DANGER RESPONSE AND BREATHING

Dr Robert Naviaux, Professor of Medicine at the University of California, suggests that it is how our mitochondria (our cells) produce energy that provides the answer to our health. Mitochondria are involved in every function of the body as our tissues and organs need energy to prevent organ failure. Chronic disease is the most obvious manifestation of long-term mitochondrial dysfunction. Dr Naviaux's research shows that as well as producing energy, our mitochondria are involved in defending the body if a threat is perceived. The more that our cells have to work in defence mode, the less energy they produce. He calls this the cell danger response (CDR) (Naviaux *et al.* 2016). The CDR means that our cells are then caught in repeating loops of incomplete recovery and are unable to fully heal. Types of threat that trigger the CDR include viruses, infections, toxins, physical injury, inflammation, poor nutrition (including excess sugar and junk food) and severe emotional stress (including trauma). If our body perceives such a threat, the CDR then comes online to maintain cell survival by putting our mitochondria into a shutdown mode. The more the mitochondria are in this defence mode, the less energy they can produce.

Mitochondria make adenosine triphosphate (ATP) as their fuel. However, if new ATP is not made because of the CDR, it takes longer for lactic acid to clear from the muscles, which results in muscle pain, especially after exercise. This may explain the severity of fatigue and PEM after activity in those with Long Covid, and also why fatigue can be delayed after too much exercise. It is therefore vital for those with Long Covid and other chronic fatigue conditions, such as post viral fatigue or ME/CFS, to rest and pace themselves after any physical or emotional activity, to give time for new ATP to be generated.

The connection between the CDR and functional breathing may lie in the link between stress, inflammation and respiratory function, because cells need oxygen in order to produce ATP. We know from Chapter 1 that when we are stressed, this results in a cascade of physiological responses, including dysfunctional breathing. Germain *et al.* (2018) explain that lack of oxygen might play an important role in chronic fatigue: 'Disturbances in circulation and provision of oxygen to tissues could underlie many symptoms of ME/CFS.'

David Systrom, a pulmonary and critical care doctor at Brigham and Women's Hospital, Boston, also studied patients with ME/CFS, an illness that bears many similarities to Long Covid. When Dr Systrom studied the mitochondrial DNA of these patients, it appeared to be normal, but after conducting muscle biopsies, he identified abnormalities deep within the mitochondria:

> In both ME/CFS and Long Covid, it's most likely that these are acquired forms of mitochondrial dysfunction, perhaps related to the initial infection itself or an auto-immune response to a virus or both. This impedes the mitochondrial machinery, but doesn't affect the DNA itself, and it means the mitochondria then fail to generate appropriate amounts of ATP to serve the needs of the muscles. (quoted in Cox 2022)

Addressing fatigue and illness effectively could involve identifying and managing the factors that trigger the CDR. This will include reducing exposure to toxins, addressing chronic infections or inflammation, implementing good nutrition, improving the gut microbiome, paying attention to the circadian rhythm and promoting cellular repair and recovery via breathing practices that encourage effective oxygenation of the cells. *Managing stress levels is obviously a big one. This is where yoga can help. Lots of functional breathing practices to regulate the breath, relaxation, gentle movement and learning to pace and stop when needed are clearly all vital pointers to healing and will help the mitochondria to recover.*

KEY POINTS

✓ Breathing functionally is key for recovery from Long Covid and fatigue-related health conditions.

✓ Breathing pattern disorders (BPDs) are common and often characterized by rapid, shallow mouth breathing.

✓ Relearning how to breathe more effectively cultivates calm, reduces stress and anxiety and increases overall wellbeing.

✓ Functional breathing involves making changes such as moving from mouth to nose breathing, and engaging the diaphragm as we breathe. These changes can feel challenging and take time and practice.

✓ Conscious awareness of breath throughout the day offers multiple chances to meditate and increase body–mind connection.

✓ Our breath is intrinsically connected to our nervous system state. When in the sympathetic nervous system (SNS) state, or the stress response, breathing is likely to be rapid and shallow. This is called hyperventilation. Slowing the exhalation engages the parasympathetic nervous system (PNS).

✓ Spending time on screen impacts our breathing pattern and disrupts functional breathing.

✓ Hyperventilation reduces levels of CO_2, which impacts delivery of oxygen to the body and brain, affecting memory and focus, and contributing to brain fog and fatigue.

✓ The cell danger response (CDR) theory proposed by Dr Robert Naviaux suggests that understanding how the mitochondria function can assist in recovery. The more our cells need to defend against threat, the less energy they produce. This impacts our ability to heal and recover from illness.

✓ Managing stress levels and understanding how stress impacts the breath helps us identify and manage factors that affect effective oxygenation at a cellular level.

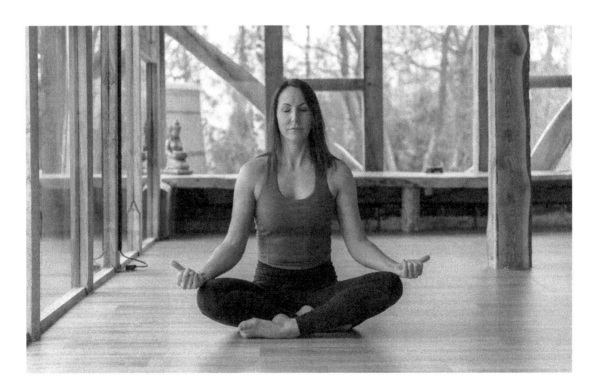

Chapter 4

BREATHING FOR RECOVERY

THE NOSE KNOWS BEST

Historically, the yogis always maintained that we should breathe through the nose. You might think, however, that mouth breathing provides more oxygen and that nose breathing means not enough air is getting to the lungs. But this is simply not the case and, contrary to popular breathing recommendations, we advise breathing *out* as well as in through the nose. In the nose versus mouth debate, the nose comes out as the winner every time, because when it comes to breathing, our mouth has no function. It is breathing through the nose that promotes better uptake of oxygen.

Studies have shown that exhaling through the mouth results in loss of heat and up to 42 per cent more water than exhaling through the nose (Svensson *et al.* 2006). This loss of heat and water can contribute to dehydration, affecting overall health and energy levels, and in addition, feelings of congestion, further perpetuating mouth breathing. This, in turn, increases BPDs.

Nasal breathing has advantages for everyone, especially for those recovering from Long Covid. An important benefit is the increased production of nitric oxide (NO), which we produce in the sinuses. NO plays a key role in regulating the cardiovascular system. It provides the advantages of being anti-microbial, anti-bacterial and, importantly, antiviral. NO increases oxygen uptake by as much as 20 per cent. It also acts as a vasodilator to the smooth muscle of the airways, opening blood vessels and preventing constriction, which makes it easier to breathe (Taneja 2020). NO also plays a role in regulating inflammation and increasing the immune response.

Research has shown that NO inhibits the replication of SARS CoV2 in a dose-dependent manner (Akaberi *et al.* 2020). Having higher levels of NO therefore gives more protection against the replication of the Covid virus. Clearly, for those experiencing Long Covid or wanting to prevent catching the virus in the first place, nasal breathing should be the only way to breathe.

BENEFITS OF NASAL BREATHING

- Nasal breathing is slower than mouth breathing. It is more challenging to breathe quickly through the nose, and so we learn to breathe more slowly. This sends calming messages, via the PNS to the brain, helping to downgrade the stress response. This has powerful benefits for anxiety, fatigue, chronic stress and pain.

- Nasal breathing adds 50 per cent more resistance to air flow, increasing the pressure in the lungs during exhalation, which simulates a lower altitude effect where the air is richer in oxygen per unit volume. This therefore increases perfusion (oxygen uptake) to the lungs.

- Efficient uptake of O2 to the cells is what we are aiming for, and the increase in lung volume caused by nasal breathing results in 10–20 per cent more uptake of O2 to the cells. Because nose breathing is slower, nasal exhalation creates a back flow of air into the lungs. The air therefore stays in the lungs for longer, and the body has more time to extract oxygen from that air.

- The inside of the nose is lined with tiny hairs called cilia. These act as filters and protect us from up to 20 billion particles of foreign matter each day.

- The nose is our very own air conditioning unit, warming and humidifying the air to the perfect temperature each time we inhale.

- Breathing through the nose stimulates the diaphragm due to the extra resistance that is needed.

- Inhaling and exhaling through the nose keeps the airways clear. Inhaling through the nose and exhaling through the mouth, however, can cause nasal congestion (Cottle 1987).

- Nose breathing takes less effort and is 22 per cent more efficient (Dallam *et al.* 2018) than mouth breathing, meaning breathing muscles don't get so tired.

- Nose breathing during sleeping is vital to reduce sleep apnea and sleep disorders, and to increase oxygenation at a time when the brain and body are recovering and replenishing. You will sleep better when you are breathing through the nose, which is why we include mouth taping in the 'Breathing and sleeping' section.

- In terms of yoga, two of the major energy channels (called *nadis* in Sanskrit) start at the nostrils, so breathing through the nose is very important for moving *prana* (energy) to the *chakras*. We look at this in more detail in the next chapter.

- Nasal breathing protects airways from inflammation.

So, we can see that nasal breathing is best, but what if we find breathing through the nose difficult?

HOW DO WE DO IT?

Many of us experience congestion, stuffy noses or allergies, or just find it difficult to switch to nasal breathing after many years of unconsciously breathing through the mouth. When we bring our awareness to the breath, however, we can begin to notice if we are mouth or nose breathing. This helps us to make changes. Remember what we said at the beginning of Chapter 1 – awareness is key.

Breath retraining can be especially problematic for those with Long Covid. Hyperventilation may have created feelings of anxiety, isolation and fear comparable to states of panic. It is essential therefore to take things slowly as we adapt to a healthier breathing pattern. If you've been a habitual mouth breather for years, the muscles of the face might be deconditioned, which means it will take time and practice to strengthen them. Therefore, we need to be gentle but also consistent to retrain our breathing patterns. Stop at any stage during the practices if you need to and allow your body to recover before starting again. We promise it will get easier!

LET'S PRACTISE: The nose unblocking technique

This technique is cited by Patrick McKeown (2015) as an effective way to temporarily increase CO_2 levels to open the nasal passages:

1. Sit comfortably and take a few slow, calm breaths.

2. Breathe in through the nose for a count of two and then exhale through the nose for a count of three.

3. Gently pinch the nose, keeping the mouth closed so the remaining air is held.

4. Slowly nod your head as you hold the nose for a few seconds. Please note that holding the breath for long periods of time during the recovery period of Long Covid can be challenging, may contribute to exhaustion and can induce feelings of panic, so please go very gently. In other words, please don't hold your breath for too long.

5. After a few seconds, breathe out through the nose slowly and begin again after two to three 'normal' breaths.

6. Repeat up to five times.

A note on breath-holding

For anyone leaning towards perfectionist or 'push/achieve' traits, please be aware that pausing the breath for long periods of time, although recommended by some breathing practitioners, will not be helpful in the long run of recovery from Long Covid, as we explained in the previous chapter. We acknowledge how difficult this can be and that you want to do anything to feel better and return to 'normal'. But this is not the time to push on through. We address this later in this book.

OTHER WAYS TO HELP UNBLOCK THE NOSE

- Natural methods of easing congestion include pressing firmly into the opposite armpit area for two minutes (Brown and Gerbarg 2012, p.21), which stimulates sensory nerves and helps to clear nasal passages.

- Sleep or sit in an upright position.

- Massage the sinuses by moving the index fingers in small circles along your brow, around your nose, under your eyes and across the cheekbones using gentle pressure and working outwards from the nose.

- Have a warm shower or bath so the humid air helps loosen any stuffy sensation.

- Saline solutions can help, perhaps alongside use of a neti pot. Using a neti pot to clear the sinuses is an ancient yogic technique and is an excellent way of preventing viruses and helping to make nasal breathing easier. If you are interested, we suggest you check in with your local yoga teacher who can show you how to do this, or look at a demonstration on YouTube.

BREATHING AND SLEEPING

Sleep can be problematic for people with Long Covid. Unfortunately, poor breathing habits go hand in hand with insomnia. However, sleep is one of the best things we can do for our recovery because it is overnight that our brains and bodies repair and reset. Good sleep improves energy, and promotes better cognitive ability, focus, memory consolidation and hormone regulation. The list goes on. We all know how we feel when we don't sleep well.

The health risks of mouth breathing at night (Summer and Rehman 2024) are not good for our sleep and so we suggest mouth taping. This is becoming widely known and is used as a way to promote more healthful sleep to assist recovery. Mouth taping also keeps us from unconsciously hyperventilating, which will interfere with deep sleep because it can trigger the stress response, raising cortisol levels.

If you wish to try sleep tape, we have the following tips and guidance:

- A small piece of tape should be placed across the mouth vertically, from the upper lip to the lower lip, about the size of a large stamp. There is no need to tape right across the mouth. We are encouraging and reminding the muscles around the mouth to relax, in order to promote nasal breathing.

- Try the taping during the day first so that you become used to the feeling of having a small piece of tape across the lips. The last thing we need at night is a nervous system on high alert because of something different, so take time when you are awake, perhaps when watching TV or pottering around the house, to get used to nasal breathing with the mouth tape on.

- It is vital to get the right tape – there is no need to reach for the gaffer tape! An inexpensive roll of micropore tape is all that is needed.

- The tape can be easily removed, but a small tip if you have facial hair is to moisten the tape with your tongue before removing to reduce the 'pull' effect on hair and skin.

LET'S PRACTISE: Increasing nitric oxide with the Humming Bee breath

Known by yogis as *brahmari* or the humming bee breath, this breathing practice was named after the sound made by a type of black Indian bee. The buzzing sound is similar to that produced by humming on an exhale. Practising this breath not only calms the mind, thus reducing agitation and anxiety, but also increases the availability of nitric oxide (NO). Humming causes air to oscillate, which, in turn, speeds up the exchange of air between the sinuses and the nasal cavity. Humming on the exhale also helps to increase the length of the exhale, which takes us out of the stress response, engages the PNS, and also helps to tone the vagus nerve. We introduced this breath in the first two chapters, but here we suggest you might like to try more repetitions, especially as you now understand the advantages of increasing NO.

1. Sit comfortably and inhale through the nose with your mouth closed.

2. As you exhale through the nose, make a 'hmmmmmmmmm' sound through closed lips.

3. As with everything we recommend, please be gentle with this practice. There's no need to force the sound on the exhalation.

4. Repeat 5–10 times, humming out the breath slowly on every out-breath.

THE TONGUE

A yoga technique known as *kechari mudra* means that you place the tip of the tongue on the soft palate towards the nasal cavity, at the roof of the mouth, keeping everything relaxed. This can be very helpful in helping to change to nasal breathing because, in mouth breathing, the tongue tends to rest on the lower palate. According to yoga, *kechari mudra* helps to increase energy and promotes balance of the whole system.

LET'S PRACTISE: *Kechari*

1. Place the tip of your tongue on the roof of your mouth, just behind the front teeth but a little further back, pointing in the direction of your nasal cavity. It takes consistent practice to do this, but you will notice that it is almost impossible to mouth breathe when the tongue is placed here.

2. Keep the tongue relaxed.

3. See if you can leave it there without thinking about this during the day.

MOVING TOWARDS A HEALTHIER BREATHING PATTERN

The average breathing rate per minute in the UK is between 12 and 18 breaths per minute (BPM) (NHS CUH 2019). Many people with Long Covid, however, have a BPM of 25 and upwards. With time and practice, you can reduce your breathing to a slower state, which we know has marked health benefits. It's very important that you don't judge yourself if you are breathing fast. Recovery takes time, and the smaller the steps the better the outcome.

Note that reducing the breathing rate to any slower than 6 BPM may actually induce further fatigue and brain fog.

SPEECH PROBLEMS AND MOUTH BREATHING

Someone who talks too fast without taking enough pauses to listen is demonstrating a hyperventilation pattern. If you are a habitual mouth breather, you may notice, as you become more aware of your breathing pattern, that you find yourself gasping when speaking, or rushing through sentences. So, we also need to consider our speech patterns when retraining the breath. Statistics demonstrate that a high number of teachers and healthcare workers have self-reported Long Covid symptoms. As well as being at the frontline of Covid, these are high-pressure professions that require numerous hours spent talking. Among many of the symptoms experienced, a feeling of needing to gasp for breath during speech is consistently demonstrated in this population. Taking steps to slow down speech, together with nasal breathing, is an important part of retraining the breath.

CHEST BREATHING

In working with hundreds of people with Long Covid and fatigue, we have observed that chest breathing is the norm, with diaphragmatic breathing often a problem. As we have seen, chest breathing also underlies many stress-related conditions, such as anxiety and fatigue.

Paradoxical breathing, where the movement of the diaphragm is reversed, may also be considered a form of trauma and chronic stress breathing. In cases of ME/CFS and Long Covid, it's not unusual to see a posture where the shoulders are hunched forward and the belly is tightly held in, which negatively impacts the diaphragm. When we take into consideration the biomechanics, societal aspects and emotional effects of trauma on the body, we can understand how our ability to use the diaphragm optimally is challenged. Unfortunately, the long-term ramifications of non-diaphragmatic movement, and the overuse of chest breathing, have very negative effects on the nervous system, which includes the heart rate, digestion and blood pressure. All of these affect our overall mental and physical health.

THE DIAPHRAGM

The diaphragm is one of the most important muscles in the body, and yet many of us don't know very much about it. It is the primary muscle for respiration and sits below the lungs, separating the chest cavity from the abdominal cavity. When inhaling, the diaphragm contracts and flattens and the chest cavity enlarges. When exhaling, it relaxes back.

The diaphragm and the surrounding area are connected to our circulatory system. Our primary muscles for stability and movement attach to the diaphragm. It is easy to see why this muscle is essential for healthy breathing, and many things can be linked to diaphragmatic dysfunction. For example, anything that overwhelms our ability to stay calm means that we may hold ourselves tightly. This limits the ability of the diaphragm to move efficiently, so that other accessory muscles compensate for respiration. This is why dysfunctional breathing is often coupled with tightness or pain to the neck (scalene muscles), chest (pectoral and intercostal muscles) and shoulders (upper trapezius and levator scapulae), as the upper ribs and chest take over when we are not utilizing the diaphragm.

LET'S PRACTISE: Moving for release

This practice helps to release the upper body muscles that are often overused if we have dysfunctional breathing.

1. Begin by sitting in an easy posture. This can be on the floor or on a chair. For some this may be cross-legged, but use comfort as your guide, ensuring you choose a position that allows your spine to be upright so that you feel at ease.

2. Focus on lifting your spine gently, visualizing the creation of space and length so that the lower ribs are free and the heart is lifted.

3. Notice your chin and the position of your head.

4. Gently draw your head into a position that feels like it is in line with the natural curves of your spine. You can do this by nodding your head up, then elongating the back of the neck. Slightly tuck the chin into the chest to keep the back of the neck long. This helps to counter-pose the common 'head forward' posture from using tech devices. Try and keep this position as you move your neck in the next sequence.

5. Start by gently rolling your shoulders a few times. Just observe if they are tight and how this movement feels, without making any judgement.

6. Look to the left, gliding the chin towards the left shoulder, keeping the chin parallel to the floor.

7. Look back to the centre, and then slowly to the right, gliding your chin towards the right shoulder, keeping your chin parallel to the floor.

8. Look back towards the centre. Repeat a few times to each side.

9. Gently take your left ear towards your left shoulder, allowing a natural opening in the right side of the neck.

10. Notice your breathing, if it is comfortable to do so. Then take your left hand and gently place it on the right side of your head so the sensation deepens.

11. Bring your head back to centre and gently take your ear towards your right shoulder.

12. Notice your breathing again, and if it is comfortable, take your right hand and gently place it on the left side of your head, allowing the left side of the neck to extend a little further. Come back to the centre.

13. Keeping the right hand on the floor if you are sitting on a mat or right knee if in a chair, lift the left arm up and near to the ear to open out the left side of the body. Keep the spine upright. Take a few breaths.

14. Lower the left hand back down.

15. Keeping the left hand on the floor or left knee, lift the right hand and bring the right arm up and near to the ear to open out the right side of the body. Take a few breaths here.

16. Lower the right hand back down. Take some resting breaths, just observing how you are feeling, without making any judgement.

17. Slowly begin to roll the shoulders upwards towards your ears, and then back, sliding the shoulder blades together, then releasing them down the back. Repeat up to five times if comfortable. Pause, take a few breaths and observe how you are.

18. Take your hands behind you, and place one hand on the opposite forearm so you are linking around the base of the spine.

19. Lean back to open up the front body and to lift the heart. If you need to, you can use blocks or books to rest your hands behind you, to manage any intensity across the collarbones and chest. This helps the front of the body to open, to free the diaphragm.

20. Return to the centre and bring your hands back to your knees.

21. Now circle your torso slowly. Imagine 'stirring' your spine as if it was a spoon in a pot of soup. Circle one way, then the other, a few times, then come back to a comfortable seated position. Pause again and observe how you are with curiosity.

22. Next, cross your hands over your chest, placing each hand on opposite shoulders.

23. With your arms hugged across your heart, focus on the breath becoming slower and lower towards the belly space. Take a few breaths here.

24. Release your arms and pause, observing how you feel.

25. Rest as much as you need to, before carrying on with your day.

> It is important to note that, for many of us, the subtle messaging we receive from our culture encourages the sense that we need to hold our abdomen in to create an 'idealized' version of our bodies. This has an adverse effect on the diaphragm. Body-based issues are often unconsciously created and conditioned from a young age. Like any habit we have adopted, this can take time to change, and so we must work gently with this area, allowing ourselves to soften and release so the diaphragm can move more effectively.

LET'S PRACTISE: Softening

1. Sit upright comfortably, or lie down.

2. Place your hands on your belly and allow your eyes to close, if that feels comfortable to do so.

3. Begin to sense the journey of the breath as it enters the nose.

4. Allow yourself to feel the rise and fall of the belly beneath your hands.

5. Please know that even if this is not happening, or you are unable to sense the movements, you can instead just imagine them happening.

6. Connect to the words 'soft', 'gentle', 'safe', 'calm' – whichever word you relate to the most.

7. Allow your mind to connect an image, quality or colour to that word.

8. With each breath, envisage this image, quality or colour at the belly, so with each rise and fall there is a sense of softening, gentleness, safety and calm.

9. Continue breathing in this way, with each inhale connecting to the word and image, quality or colour, and allowing each exhale to take care of itself.

10. Don't exaggerate any movement in the belly by breathing too deeply, but keep the breath slow and subtle if you can.

More about the function of the diaphragm

When we are using the diaphragm properly, we are creating more space for the breath within the lungs. The two lower ribs then expand laterally (outwards), and this helps to draw more air down, encouraging a more effective gaseous exchange. The lower area of the lungs is also where our calming receptors reside, which engages the PNS branch. Conversely, when we breathe from the chest, we stimulate the upper nerve receptors in the lungs, creating arousal to the SNS (stress response). It's like a circle – the stress response makes us breathe faster through the mouth and upper chest, ready to fight or flee, but if we continue to breathe in this way when the stress has passed, we will continue to be held in a stress pattern. *To break this cycle, we need to retrain our breathing pattern so that we engage the diaphragm and breathe more slowly, through the nose.*

LET'S PRACTISE: Diaphragmatic breathing

Please note, you need to lie on your back for this exercise. If you can't yet do this, please move on.

1. Lie down comfortably on your back.

2. Place your hands on your belly and allow your eyes to close, if you would like to.

3. Begin to sense the breath as it enters the nose, if you are able to.

4. Allow yourself to feel the movement of the belly beneath your hands.

5. You may wish to place a weighted soft object on your abdominal area in order to feel the rise and fall with each breath – we recommend a small, weighted pillow, no heavier than 2kg, or a small bag of rice.

6. Encourage each breath to be slow, smooth and low, allowing the belly to move a little each time you inhale and exhale.

7. Continue to breathe in this way for a few minutes.

8. Please note that if you feel uncomfortable or if there is pain, you should stop the practice and return to your normal breathing rhythm. Every day is different, and tomorrow is a new day to explore this practice again.

BALANCED BREATHING

Balanced breathing, sometimes known as coherent resonant breathing, involves a rate of approximately 6 BPM with an even inhalation and exhalation. The average inhale is for 6 seconds and the exhale of 6 seconds. However, don't let this put you off – we are starting much more gently here!

We encourage you to begin gradually with this practice and not to get too hung up on the exact number of counts until you are comfortable. You are building up to this ratio over a period of time. The aim is for a balanced inhalation and exhalation to regulate the nervous system. An inhale and exhale of 5–6 counts is something to work towards, and most people with Long Covid can't breathe this slowly. Please don't put pressure on yourself to get there too quickly. In the beginning, we recommend starting with a count of 2–3 as you inhale and exhale, taking your time to adjust. For children we don't recommend this practice at all, as their lung capacity is too small.

Clinical reports demonstrate that when we breathe with an even inhale and exhale, we improve biomarkers of health such as heart rate variability (HRV) (Steffen *et al.* 2021). Coherent, balanced breathing harmonizes and synchronizes all the systems of the body so that we exert less effort and we soothe the nervous system. In particular, this breath is effective for those experiencing PTSD and depression (Brown and Gerbarg 2012). This method of breathing has been shown to have the following benefits:

- Increases the response and activity of the PNS

- Reduces the breathing rate in general, significantly lowering symptoms of anxiety

- Helps to alter the brain wave pattern, so we enter what is often referred to as 'flow state'. This breathing rate has also been indicated in prayer, *mantra* and meditative states. Many cultures and religions consequently have the same breathing pattern as the coherent breath.

YOGA AND BALANCED BREATHING

In yoga, *samana* is a type of *prana*, or energy. We refer to coherent, or balanced, breathing as *samana* breathing. *Samana* breathing alleviates agitation and restlessness while reviving us from feelings of fatigue, lethargy and sluggishness. This type of breathing fosters a sense of balance and tranquillity, leading us to a state characterized by the *guna* of *sattva*. In contemporary terms, we can liken this to the body's state of homeostasis, where all body systems are in equilibrium, promoting harmony within body, mind and spirit.

LET'S PRACTISE: Balanced breathing

1. Sit or lie down and make yourself as comfortable as you can, with support from cushions or bolsters and whatever else you need.

2. You may wish to place your hands on your belly and to close your eyes.

3. Begin to breathe gently, inhaling and exhaling through the nose if you can.

4. As you tune in to the breath, start by counting to three or four as you inhale, using the same count as you exhale. If this is too challenging, you could start with a count of two.

5. A reminder that if this ratio does not work for you at present, reduce to even lower, and gradually increase your count, when you feel ready. Try not to be goal-oriented, but go gently and use this opportunity as a practice of self-compassion and acceptance (more on this later in the book).

6. Over time, you can build up to a count of six on the inhale and six on the exhale. Be aware that this might take several months, so don't be hard on yourself if this seems a big ask. Just do what is comfortable for now.

7. No effort should be required for this practice. Let both breaths be gentle and without exertion. If you are struggling in any way, lower the count. If you aim for a balanced and even inhalation and exhalation, then you are breathing coherently.

8. Continue to breathe in this way for as long as is comfortable. You can slowly, over time (we are talking weeks and months, not days), begin to increase the length of this practice to 10 minutes or more if accessible, but begin with 2–3 minutes maximum until you feel comfortable to gently increase the time.

Tip: You may like to practise this in bed at night, before you go to sleep.

POSTURAL CONSIDERATIONS AND RESTORATIVE BREATHING

Prone positioning, or lying on the stomach, has long been used in intensive care units to address acute respiratory distress (Sud *et al.* 2014). Prone positioning, or proning, as it is also known, helps to improve the amount of oxygen uptake, because lying in this position prevents the heart and stomach from pressing on the lungs. Consequently, we include some prone postures in the yoga practices in the book. We also always give the option of resting on the front when coming to a lying position, in case it is easier for breathing.

In all our practices we suggest finding a resting position that best suits your needs. Although the classical posture in traditional yoga is *savasana* (relaxation pose) on the back, this may be totally unsuitable for you at this time. And that is okay. As you learn to listen to your body's needs, use this as an opportunity to find what works best for you.

For Long Covid, we suggest the Crocodile position to assist optimal breathing, if you would like to experiment with lying on your front. This allows a sense of feedback for diaphragmatic breathing, and is also a powerful method of relieving anxiety and tension in the body. However, as with all practices, they are only restful if they are comfortable. We advise placing support or padding underneath you if there is discomfort.

LET'S PRACTISE: Crocodile

1. Lie on your belly, placing whatever support you need underneath you.

2. Using your hands, create a pillow beneath your forehead with one hand on top of the other, so your forehead is resting on the back of your hands.

3. If more support is needed to create space for the nose, please use a pillow or cushion as required. You can also experiment with having your head to one side, with arms beside the body.

4. Focus on the breath, if that feels okay for you.

5. As you inhale, feel the belly slightly press towards the floor, and on each exhalation, feel the pressure release. Focus on awareness of this slight pressure against the floor on the inhale, and the softening of the belly on the exhale.

6. Breathe gently and softly, allowing a sense of gentle expansion throughout the body with each breath. There is no need to force anything or to breathe too deeply.

7. Now be aware of breathing into your back. Take a few breaths, keeping your awareness of the breath here.

8. Feel that you are breathing and expanding into the back with every inhale. Even if you can't sense this, just visualize the breath expanding into the back. Focus on a smooth, slow, quiet and subtle breath, directing the breath low in the body towards the belly and around the back. If it's helpful, visualize the breath as filling the back with light.

9. Continue to breathe in this way for as long as is comfortable.

Precautions: Pregnancy and anyone experiencing intense discomfort when lying on the front. If this is the case, try lying on the side, supported with any cushions and padding to make yourself comfortable.

OTHER POSTURES TO TRY

Elevating the legs can have a profound effect on our health. Yogis have been doing this for years because it has many benefits including calming the nervous system. Leg elevation is a way of improving blood flow. This is because, unlike our arteries, veins use tiny valves to assist circulation, and the contraction of the surrounding muscles assists this movement back towards the heart. When sitting or standing, oxygen-depleted blood must work against gravity in order to return to the heart. Elevating the legs places them above the level of the heart, thus assisting blood circulation more efficiently.

A lesser known but very important benefit is that raising the legs helps the glymphatic system. This is part of the lymph system of the brain and is a second filtration process, which removes unwanted pathogens, filtering the metabolic waste that accumulates every day from the nervous system. Therefore, elevating the legs can assist with oxygenation and detoxification of the whole body, which may help with brain fog and energy.

LET'S PRACTISE: Elevated legs

1. Ensure you have appropriate support for your body, maybe having a cushion under your head.

2. You may wish to use a wall, a chair or sofa, or perhaps a stack of cushions, to keep the legs comfortably raised.

3. Relaxation is key, so take a few moments to wiggle into the cosiest position for your body as you raise your legs higher than your head, while keeping your upper body relaxed on the floor. If you are using a wall, a tip is to come into the wall sideways, and swing round gently to help raise the legs to the optimum position. If you are using a chair, try to have a 45-degree angle between the body and legs.

4. Focus on breathing slowly and calmly, moving your awareness slowly from your feet to your head on the inhale, and from your head to your feet on the exhale. If you don't want to follow the breath or the visualization, just relax.

5. Rest here for 10–15 minutes, or as long as it feels good.

6. To come out from this position, hug your knees towards your chest and roll to one side.

7. Take time to rest on your side, before spiralling up very slowly, to sit in a comfortable position.

Precautions: Laying flat on the back with legs raised can be problematic for those experiencing the following (please check with your health professional if you are unsure): pregnancy, glaucoma or any eye pressure problems, untreated high blood pressure.

GUIDANCE AND PRECAUTIONS

When we look at how we should be breathing, it's very important to understand what we need to avoid, because certain breathing techniques can make conditions such as Long Covid or ME/CFS worse.

- Breath holding for more than a couple of seconds should not be implemented, unless recovery is greatly improved. A controlled pause is recommended by many breathing resources such as the Buteyko method and Wim Hof. We believe these may indeed be therapeutic, but are not for those with Long Covid unless well recovered.

- A reminder that the first *yama* (code of practice) in the *Yoga Sutras* is the Sanskrit word *ahimsa*. The meaning of this is non-violence, and this starts with the attitude towards oneself. In other words, we should always aim to practise with kindness and compassion. This particularly applies to our breathing practice – nothing should be forced or rushed.

- Bringing awareness to the breath and changing breathing patterns can, if not done gently, be a cause of anxiety as well as encouraging physiological change, which can induce unwelcome sensations including dizziness. Therefore, we have to take baby steps and work slowly.

- People with Long Covid may have entrenched poor breathing patterns, and pre-existing conditions such as asthma and/or anxiety will exacerbate their symptoms. Work gently and encourage awareness of the first signs of panic or anxious thoughts, so that you or your client can stop or focus on their Safe Resource.

- Ensure you work within a window of their personal tolerance – nothing should be prescriptive. In other words, this work should be client-led.

- Practices for anxious, breathless students should begin with neck and shoulder mobility to promote easing of the accessory muscles often used as compensation for breathing (Brown and Gerbarg 2012).

- Coherent breathing (balanced inhalation and exhalation) can be a challenge for those with reduced lung capacity. Gradual progression is advised, along with the practice of self-compassion, especially for those experiencing anxiety, as explained in the practice above. This is very important – nothing should be forced. Build up slowly.

- Shutting one nostril may induce a panic response in some people, so we should avoid teaching the Alternate Nostril breath as a physical practice. Our advice would be to instead visualize the air entering and leaving alternate nostrils.

- For more guidance and precautions of breathing for Long Covid, please also see the Guidance section at the beginning of the book.

KEY POINTS

✓ Nasal breathing is best for many reasons, one of which is the production of nitric oxide (NO), which plays a key role in regulating the cardiovascular system and oxygen uptake.

✓ Nasal breathing helps to slow the breath, assisting in down-regulation of the nervous system and reducing stress.

✓ If nasal breathing is difficult, we can try the nose unblocking technique. The more we breathe through the nose, the easier nasal breathing will become.

✓ Sleep is a time when we replenish and recover. Breathing well at night is vital. We recommend sleep tape to re-establish nasal breathing at night if you are a mouth breather. Please follow the guidance in the chapter.

✓ Humming helps to increase NO levels and can increase feelings of calm.

✓ The diaphragm is one of the most important muscles in the body and is the primary muscle for respiration.

✓ If we have dysfunctional breathing, we may over-engage the muscles of the neck and upper shoulders, which can become tight and tense.

✓ Retraining our breathing patterns and encouraging effective movement of the diaphragm takes time and should be approached gently.

✓ Coherent breathing aims for a balanced inhale and exhale to harmonize body systems and soothe the nervous system.

✓ It's important to be gentle with yourself when retraining the breath. Working with a trained breathing coach, therapist or yoga therapist can be useful.

Chapter 5

HOW *PRANAYAMA* CAN INCREASE ENERGY AND WELLBEING

In the *Yoga Sutras*, Patanjali explains that yoga happens when the mind is calm and quiet. Yoga is described in the ancient texts as 'union' or 'to yoke'. This means the bringing together of the real self (something we cover later in the book when we talk about the need to be authentic) with something that is greater than us, and which we might call universal intelligence, divine mystery or even God. We can also just call it Life, by which we mean that yoga can lead to the understanding that we are not separate from anything. The point here is that health challenges give us the time and space to question what life is really about. Patanjali also explains that the goal of yoga is freedom (Desikachar 2003, *Yoga Sutras* 4.34). We may understand this as freedom from the stories and agitation of the mind and a complete acceptance of life as it is, as it unfolds in each moment. This is a hard one, because when things are not going as we hoped, acceptance is very difficult because the mind will continue to spin (often negative) stories. Yet it is in this deepest non-resistance to our experience, even when we are in pain and chronically tired, that we may find the gold of existence. We hope the rest of the book unfolds these ideas. But ultimately, what we are saying is that yoga can help us to reframe our suffering as a portal to peace.

One of the defining features of Long Covid is lack of energy. A defining feature of yoga, however, is that it is *about* energy. So, yoga is very different from conventional systems of movement and exercise and offers an effective route back to wellness because of the philosophy of *prana*, which means, roughly translated, life force energy. *Prana* is also considered to be the link between spirit and matter (Feuerstein 1990). For the purpose of this book, we can think of *prana* as being something that flows continuously, filling us and keeping us alive. It is essential vitality and is also known as a system of light that nourishes and sustains us on every level. When *prana* leaves the body there is no life. According to Vedic science, *prana* makes up the whole of the manifest universe and evolved from the divine principle of creation, the first sound of which was 'Om', which created *prana*. It is said that divinity resides wherever *prana* flows. *Mantra*, or certain Sanskrit sounds when chanted, works to move *prana* and is said to influence all structures of the body and to protect the mind. We cannot work with *prana* effectively without *mantra*, which is considered in yoga therapy to be the power behind healing. Therefore, sound is included as an option in many of the practices, because it can be of immense benefit in Long Covid. (And in Chapter 2 you may remember we explored how sound helps to regulate vagal tone.)

Quantum mechanics confirms what the ancient yogis knew: we are made of energy and are actually a mass of vibrating particles (Grey 2019), because everything is made of sequences of energy. Atoms are part of this. There is energy in even the tiniest fragment of the universe and these are in constant motion. The theory of relativity shows that mass is not only a solid substance (as it appears to us) but is a form of energy. If, through yoga, we can unlock the code of how to move energy more effectively, then we have the secret to wellbeing and health. We are claiming that this may indeed be possible. We start by understanding *prana* and how we can use it to our advantage.

As we breathe, we bring *prana* into the system via something called *nadis*. These are subtle energy channels (allegedly 72,000 of them) that feed our energy centres or *chakras*. Every *chakra* is a centre for *prana*, and because the *chakras* are so important for health, most of the practices that we share in this book are based around them. The nature of *prana* is to move, and as it enters through two major *nadis* (*ida* and *pingala*) at the nostrils, it spirals along a path called the *susumna nadi*, which runs parallel to the spine. There are both material and subtle sources of *prana*. The material elements include things such as fresh whole foods, a beautiful environment, good connection with uplifting people, sunshine, nature and pure spring water. Subtle sources of *prana* include love, beauty and creativity. *The most important source of* prana *according to yoga therapy is the breath.* This is very interesting because, as we have already seen in the previous chapters, how we breathe is profoundly affected by our state of health and vice versa. The breath and *prana* are so closely related that when our breathing is impacted by something (such as shock, trauma, chronic stress or illness), our vitality is also affected. *Consequently, huge emphasis in yoga and in this book is put on* pranayama. *Pranayama* is an energetic practice that influences our *prana* and our health. *Pranayama* means the extension of breath, of the vital life force, and describes certain breathing techniques that we use in yoga to help improve wellbeing and vitality. *Pranayama* is conscious and regulated breathing. In Chapters 3 and 4 we looked at some science-based breathing techniques for Long Covid. Now we are going to see how these relate to the healing effects of yoga breathing.

All the practices in this book have an element of *pranayama*. In yoga therapy, *pranayama* is considered the chief way of rejuvenating the body and also of managing the movement of the mind. (You may remember we started the book by explaining that the mind can be our source of healing, or it can work against us. We want it to do the former.) Certain techniques such as prolonging the hold after exhalation (not recommended for

Long Covid until recovered, as explained previously) are considered to extend life as well as to increase energy. Working with the breath is always an individual approach, helping someone from where they are at, and remembering that too much interference or anything complicated may heighten anxiety in someone who has difficulty in breathing. Yoga teachers and therapists should work at the pace of the student and consider how they are and what their constitution is. As we saw in the last chapter, someone may initially find it difficult to breathe through the nose, or be unable to engage the diaphragm. In a *pranayama* practice we are leading someone towards breathing more slowly, through the nose and with a smooth, controlled exhalation. Ultimately, we want the breath to be subtle. We love the expression used by Robin Rothenberg (2019), 'Slow and low', as this gives something to aim for. We work towards this in increments – something known as *krama* in yoga – and we take our time to get there, especially because, when we change the breathing pattern, this may initially seem challenging. Therefore, we always offer choice, and we never force someone to change their breathing suddenly, but let them set the pace.

The thesis of *pranayama* is that it softens and releases tensions in the system. In yogic philosophy it is considered that *prana* is always there, but it becomes restricted if 'knots' form. These energetic knots are known in Sanskrit as *granthis*. So, if you feel ill or exhausted, this means that there is a restriction in your system preventing the healthy flow of *prana*. Covid is one example of how we may get into an unhealthy pattern of breathing, which then causes a restriction. Using another example, if you shut down your emotions because of trauma, tension then becomes trapped, causing an energy block. This is often unconscious. It is therefore very important that we process our feelings effectively, otherwise they remain confined, depleting our vitality. Until recently, in our culture expressing emotions was considered unacceptable. But this can lead to a disconnection from our emotional self, and so we react to life with a lot of mental problem solving. As far as yoga is concerned, if we don't feel our emotions, energy can't move, the mind becomes increasingly agitated or depressed, and the whole system becomes exhausted. These are just examples of how *granthis* can cause energy to become stuck. When we become chronically ill it is very helpful to look at our whole being because *yoga doesn't separate us into just physical or mental, mind or body. It sees us as a union of physical, energy, mind, emotional and spiritual, all of which interact within our environment.* A yoga practice is therefore about creating space in the system so that the *granthis* can soften and all these layers of our being can come into balance.

The *panca maya* model (often referred to as the *pancha kosha*), as described in the *Taittiriya Upanishad*, explains the human being as being made up of five interconnected dimensions or layers. These five layers consist of: (1) *annamaya*, the physical body; (2) *pranamaya*, the energetic body; (3) *manomaya*, the mind; (4) *vijnanamaya*, our higher mind such as our intuition, wisdom and deeper states of consciousness; and (5) *anandamaya*, sometimes translated as our bliss or spiritual body, and closest to our atman or true self. Wellbeing is said to arise when all five of these dimensions are integrated and balanced.

The *panca maya* is an integral part of yoga therapy, in that a therapist would always consider which layer needs to be addressed first, and then prescribe the appropriate practice. *Granthis* can occur at any of these dimensions, and disruption in one layer will affect all the others. For example, we may have a problem with mental health (the *manomaya*), which eventually affects the posture and health of the physical body (*annamaya*), or we may have a challenge with the breath (*pranamaya*), which might make the mind (*manomaya*) very agitated. In yoga therapy, we choose the appropriate tool such as *mantra*, *pranayama* and certain postures to help create space and integration of these different dimensions. This helps *prana* to flow more effectively, which encourages a state of healing. Using another example, if left unacknowledged, trapped emotions and distress eventually affect the mental (*manomaya*) and physical dimensions (*annamaya*) of the *panca maya*. Therefore, in a *pranayama* practice, we work gently to help reduce *granthis* in all layers of being to bring about coherence.

THE FIVE *PRANAS*

There are five important types of *prana* and five more minor ones. These are also known as the *maha vayu*, or great winds. Here, we are concerned with the first three major *pranas* as they are most relevant when understanding how we practise yoga to encourage healing for Long Covid and fatigue. The first of these, *prana* itself, is associated with the inhalation and the area around the chest, upper back and heart. It is an upward-flowing energy, linked to our thoughts and emotions, because *prana* is always associated with the quality of the mind. It is about nourishment, and it's said that where *prana* flows, the mind will go, and vice versa. This is one of the reasons we bring focused attention in our *pranayama* practice to how the breath is, or to parts of the body, together with visualization practices. However, this first type of *prana* can be too stimulating for those with chronic illness, which is why certain breathing techniques such as breath holds or *kapalabhati* (which focuses on a rapid inhalation) should be avoided.

The second type of energy is called *apana* and relates to our exhalation. *Apana* is associated with the lower part of the body and is a downward-flowing movement. It also correlates to the lower *chakras*, which is what we want to balance when working with Long Covid (there is more explanation of why this is in the next chapter). *Apana* provides space for elimination. If a person is slow and heavy, for example, they may have too much *apana*. In yoga it is considered vital to release what is superfluous so that *prana* can move. An analogy would be that if you bought a house, you wouldn't bring in new furniture without cleaning the house first and removing the old stuff, because the house would otherwise become cluttered and dirty, and it would be difficult to move around. Likewise, with the energy of *apana*, we want to release and detoxify what is in excess, so that the incoming *prana* can flow more effectively. The elimination of *apana* relates to our food, faecal matter, urine and sweat, as well as to our experiences, emotions and opinions. For example, if we hold on to an idea of how life was before we became ill, then *apana* is ineffective and we may feel sluggish, depressed and tired. It is therefore important to look at what we are consuming on all levels. Are we looking at social media too much? Are we addicted to the negative effects of watching the news on TV? Are we trying to do and achieve too much? Even constantly chasing self-help (books, workshops, summits, supplements, support groups and so on) can lead to overwhelm, and we need to let go of the chase. So *apana* – the energy of detoxification – isn't just about letting go on the physical level; it's about releasing toxic matter at every layer of our being (the *panca maya*). We want to let go, if we can, of all our ideas about the past, so that new circumstances can arise, otherwise we are creating an energy knot (*granthi*). The good news is that we can create space with the appropriate *pranayama* practice to help this energetic waste to be released.

Because *apana* is associated with the out-breath, we put a lot of importance on a smooth exhalation in yoga therapy, especially when working with stress and fatigue conditions such as Long Covid. Interestingly, if we want to come out of the stress response, we can do this by making the exhalation longer than the inhalation for a few breaths. In terms of yoga, this is implementing the energy of *apana*.

The third type of prana is called *samana* and relates to the area around the navel. *Samana* has the quality of equilibrium and is the meeting point of *prana* and *apana*. It is about what we assimilate and digest – not just our food, but all of our experiences. Do we grasp at something, for example, or are we able to process our life circumstances effectively before we move on? In this way we are not bypassing or denying our emotions. We can think of this as energy in motion. Healthy diaphragmatic breathing helps with this type of energy and a *samana pranayama* practice would consist of an even inhalation and exhalation. This describes the coherent breath from the previous chapter, which is a very important healing practice for those with Long Covid.

LET'S PRACTISE: *Apana*, the releasing energy

Please note that in a yoga practice, combining breath and movement can be a more effective way of introducing *pranayama* if someone is too anxious to focus just on the breath. In the following practice, we work with *apana* by incorporating movement, breathing and *mantra*. Please remember that everything is optional, so if you don't want to chant, that's fine.

1. Lie down or sit comfortably. Take a few moments to arrive in your body. Notice how you are. How is your body? How are you feeling emotionally? See if you can notice your state of being without judgement. Is there any pain? Is the mind calm or agitated?

Allow everything to be as it is, accepting everything as it is without labelling it as good or bad. If you can, bring a sense of compassion to your current experience.

2. Relax your jaw. Bring your awareness to your eyes. Fatigue can be felt here, so take a moment or two to soften your gaze. Rub your palms together and gently place them over your eyes, inviting the eyes to relax back into the eye sockets. Explore the warmth of the palms. Experiment with opening and closing your eyes. Keeping your gaze soft, look around your space. If comfortable, close your eyes.

3. Take your awareness to your breath. Without judgement – just observe. Is the breath slow or fast? Is it coming more from the upper chest or belly? Are you breathing through your mouth or nose? As you observe, see if you can be curious. Invite the breath to slow down. Observe the difference between the inhalation and exhalation. If you can, begin to focus on the exhalation, so the inhale is free. Allow the out-breath to be long and smooth. Let your breath be quiet, if possible.

4. Take one hand and place it on your heart and one on your belly. Let the breath move down into the lower hand if possible, so that the hand on the heart is relatively still. Spend a few moments feeling the rise and fall of the hand on the belly. Don't force the breath, think of the breath as being slow, low and quiet. If watching the breath makes you uncomfortable or anxious, just feel the movement of the hand, or bring your awareness to your feet.

5. Can you breathe through your nose? The practice in Chapter 4 may have helped you build up to this. If not, don't worry. Just sit quietly, focusing on a soft exhalation for a few minutes. If discomfort arises, come back to your normal breathing rhythm.

6. We are going to introduce sound, or *mantra*, which can help with the exhalation and the energy of *apana*. The ancient yogis said that the appropriate vibration through sound helps to pacify disease and clear away impurities. You might like to try, with lips together, just humming the breath out on the exhalation for up to five breaths. Or you might like to try a *mantra*: 'Om [pause]. Apana namaha.' The meaning of this is: 'I surrender to the exhalation and to the energy of elimination.' You can chant just once or up to five times. Or you might like to chant in English: 'I let go.' Choose whichever version you like. When you have finished, pause and observe how you are.

7. Inhaling, open your arms out wide to the sides. On the exhalation, cross your arms over your chest and give yourself a hug. Repeat this slowly, two or three times, with the movement following the breath as you inhale to open the arms and exhale to hug. Now pause and take a few breaths, with the arms crossed over the heart and with your eyes closed, if that feels comfortable.

8. Pause and tune in to your whole system: mind, body and emotions. Observe how you are feeling. Can you bring your focus to the still point after the exhalation?

9. Next, drop your hands to your knees. Take five slow breaths, focusing on your exhalation being longer than your inhalation. Then pause, coming back to your normal breathing rhythm, and observe the effects on your whole being: body, breath, energy, mind, emotions.

10. If you are sitting, come down to lying on your back with your knees bent. (It's also fine to remain sitting if you have any breathing difficulties and can't lie on your back.) Take a moment or two to adjust your position as you transition to lying. Have some support under your head. Very slowly, roll the head from side to side. Then centre your head. Very gently, roll the shoulders, experiencing them against the floor. (You can also do this from sitting.) Bring your awareness to your back and cultivate the idea of the Earth supporting you as you soften everything down. Feel yourself releasing on every exhalation as you relax into your support. Think of the spine as a plumb line with the right and left sides of the back softening around this centre line. Let go of your shoulders. Relax your jaw.

11. Bring awareness to your breath. Take your hands to the belly and notice the soft rise and fall of the hands as you breathe slowly and gently through the nose. If following the breath makes you feel uncomfortable, use your Safe Resource.

12. Gently bring the knees over the belly, perhaps lifting one knee first, then another. Hold around the knees. You are now going to move with the breath.

13. Inhaling, let the knees move away from you, straightening your arms. As you exhale, bring the knees in towards the belly. If it's challenging to coordinate the movement with the breath, just do what feels right. Listen to your body and honour how it feels. If you are sitting, you can visualize these next movements.

14. As you move with the breath, bring your awareness to your back. Feel the pressure gently increase against your support as your knees come in towards the body on the exhalation.

15. Bringing the knees together, begin to circle the knees apart with the breath. Inhale, gently push the knees away from you and open the knees wide apart. As you exhale, bring the knees towards the belly and then back in together. Repeat a few times so that you are circling the knees together and apart. Then invite the knees to circle in the opposite direction. As you do this, bring your awareness to your hips. Then bring your awareness to your back, noticing the massaging effect as you circle your hips and knees.

16. Drop your feet to the floor and rest with knees bent or legs straight. Take some time to observe the effect of the practice on your whole being. Allow the mind to become quiet. Consider, 'What is it I need to let go of?' Because this is a reflective question, it doesn't require an answer. Some ideas might be: 'To let go of control', 'To let go of

making decisions based around fear', 'To make future decisions based on love and not anxiety' or 'To let go of "doing" all the time and to put my health first'.

17. Focus on what nourishment you might bring into your life. This could be: 'To be a friend to myself', 'To be more authentic and to speak up for myself' or 'To connect with joy whenever possible'.

18. Now think of what brings you strength. Focus on the feeling of that quality in your heart. Stay for a moment or two, visualizing this symbol of strength – what it is that makes you feel stronger. (Ideas are a pet, a loved one, a tree, a place in nature, a mountain.)

19. Inhale and then exhale for two breaths, visualizing this symbol of strength at your feet. Then take two breaths to your knees, two breaths to your hips, two breaths to the belly, two breaths to the heart, two breaths to the throat and finally two breaths to the top of the head. On each inhalation, visualize the quality of your symbol of strength coming into the body.

20. Rest for at least five minutes.

LET'S PRACTISE: *Krama* breath

This practice incorporates an inhale, then a short pause, then another inhale, then an exhale and pause, and then an exhale. This way of breathing in steps is called *krama* in Sanskrit and may be easier for those with Long Covid who may find breathing in and out difficult. You can apply the *krama* to the inhale, the exhale, or both – experiment and see what works for you. As always, if you find this difficult, please leave this practice out. It will be easy for some and more challenging for others. It's best to practise this from sitting.

1. Inhale a little and pause, then inhale again, feeling your ribs expand outwards. If it helps, you may like to place your hands around your ribcage so that you are breathing into your hands, fingers pointing inwards around the lower ribs and thumbs around the back, to help feel this outward expansion from the in breath.

2. Exhaling, hum the breath out, drawing the navel into the spine. Pause, then exhale and hum again. Feel the hands gently come a little way together as the ribs relax.

3. Now breathe normally for three in and out breaths. Then repeat steps 1 and 2 three to five times.

4. Relax, just observing the effect of the practice on your whole being.

LET'S PRACTISE: Filling the body with
prana and light – a longer practice

The ancient teachings tell us that *prana* is light and this practice is about moving *prana* around the body.

1. From sitting, observe how you are at all levels of being, as if you were noticing the weather pattern. Be curious about your body, mind and emotions. Become aware of your breath. If comfortable, allow the breath to slow down and to be a little lower in the body.

2. Roll your shoulders slowly three times with the breath, inhaling to lift towards the ears and exhaling as they lower, drawing the shoulder blades towards each other.

3. Inhale. As you exhale, take your left ear towards your left shoulder. Inhale and centre. Exhale and take the right ear toward the right shoulder. Inhale and centre. Repeat twice more to each side.

4. Inhale, then on the exhalation roll the head to look over the right shoulder. Inhale and centre the head. Exhaling, look over your left shoulder. Inhale and centre. Repeat twice more to each side.

5. Take one hand to the heart and one to the belly, breathing into the hand at the belly. Breathe through the nose if you can. Don't judge yourself if you can't, just work with acceptance or even compassion of how you are. Take up to five breaths here.

6. Bring the palms together over the heart. Inhaling, circle the arms out to the sides and up into a prayer position (palms together) above your head. Exhaling, bring the palms slowly back down in time with the out-breath, back to the heart. Repeat three times. Then reverse the movement so you are circling in the opposite direction three times. Pause and observe how you are.

7. Become aware of the area around the eyes and soften. Soften your hearing. Release your jaw. Relax around your throat and softly lift the ribs and the heart. Visualize breathing into your back, gently drawing the navel to the spine on the exhale for five breaths. Then come back to your normal breathing rhythm. Observe if anything has changed.

8. Sit quietly for a moment or two, visualizing that you are like a mountain, rising up from your hips. Feel a sense of solidity and the strength of your mountain. Feel your feet on the floor.

9. Take the hands around the lower ribcage. Inhale into the hands. Exhale and squeeze softly, as if you were squeezing a balloon very gently. Open your mouth and make a 'shhh' sound as you exhale. Try this for five breaths.

10. Now inhale through the nose, as if you were sipping in the air in steps. So, inhale and

pause, inhale again, pause and inhale. (If two sips is enough, stop there.) 'Shhh' the air out of your mouth as you exhale.

11. Take your hands to your knees. Inhale, and lift the arms out to the sides, then up so the arms are parallel to the ears. Exhale and lower the arms, finishing with the hands on the knees, humming them down on the exhale. Repeat two to five times, depending on your energy levels.

12. Rest for a few breaths. Take the hands into prayer *mudra* over the heart. Inhale and take the arms out to the side like a cross. Exhaling, bring the palms together over the heart as you chant 'Om shanti, shanti, shanti' or 'Peace, peace, peace'. If you don't want to chant, you can hum the breath out instead, or just exhale without sound. Repeat three to five times.

13. Pause and observe the sense of peace created by the chant. Breathe in a sense of security and safety into the heart on the inhalation, if that feels comfortable. Or you might like to visualize breathing in a sense of light to the heart. Relax on the out-breath, allowing the exhale to be slightly longer than the inhalation. Focus on encouraging the out-breath to be long and smooth if you are able to. If not, that's also fine.

14. Take your fingers to the back of the skull and gently circle and then pull the fingers apart, to create space at the base of the cranium.

15. Relax the hands back to the lap. Take a few breaths, just observing the effect of the practice so far on mind, body, emotions and breath, without any judgement.

16. Visualize the world, about the shape of a large football, hovering in front of you. Observe the beauty of the oceans and the green of the forests.

17. Develop a sense of deep love and gratitude for our planet and your life here. Imagine that you are surrounding the world in front of you with love and also compassion. If you can't find these qualities for now, visualize healing light around the world.

18. Remember that you are not separate from the world or from nature. Cultivate a sense of peace for yourself, however you are, right here in this moment. Even for your symptoms and any difficulties, see if you can bring compassion and love to them. If this is too much, see if you can at least accept where you are at.

19. Breathe in a sense of light, or *prana*, into your heart on the inhale. As you exhale, send the light out to the image of the world in front of you. Encourage a longer exhale and gradually lengthen the out-breath until it is twice as long as the inhale, visualizing light covering the image of the world. If you can't extend the out-breath, that's okay.

20. Return to normal breathing. Remember that light always overcomes darkness and that within you is perfect light. Just focus on a sense of light within you.

21. As we bring in light, we must be prepared to face our shadows. This means that all our feelings are welcome, even those of anger, anxiety, agitation, resentment, fear and shame. These are the parts of us that are more hidden, but they need to be embraced, too, in order to bring about healing. If you observe any shadow emotion rising now in the space that has been created by the practice, bring a sense of deep acceptance to whatever is arising. Remember, you can focus on your Safe Resource at any time.

22. Take your hands to your heart again. Inhale and open your arms up and out to the sides, parallel to the floor. As you exhale, bring your hands together over your heart, with the idea of gathering gentle sunlight to the heart on the out-breath. Repeat 3–5 times. Pause and observe a sense of stillness.

23. With your hands in prayer at your heart, inhale and take the right arm to the side, following the hand with your gaze. Exhale the hand back to the heart as you chant 'Om shanti, shanti, shanti'. (As always, you have the option to chant 'Peace, peace, peace' if you prefer, or to hum or just breathe out without chanting.) Then inhaling, take the left arm out to the left, following the hand with your gaze. Inhale and chant the left hand back to the heart. Repeat up to three times on each side.

24. Sit quietly and observe your state of being at all levels – mind, body, emotions and energy. Allow everything to be as it is, having a sense of faith and trust that by surrendering to every moment and to life, things will be fine. All is well.

25. Now become aware of your hands. Wriggle your fingers. Feel the support under your bottom and your feet. Take some time to sit quietly before returning to your day.

LET'S PRACTISE: Creating space for *prana*

This practice is about creating space in the whole being – the *panca maya*. All of us have constrictions on some level. These are *granthis* that can occur at any dimension of our being – body, breath, mind or emotions. When we soften and create space, *prana* can start to flow and healing can take place.

1. Come into a comfortable sitting position. Notice the body, then the breath. Observe how you are at this moment.

2. Observe the space around you. Next, be aware of space in your body, space between the ribs, space in the joints. See if you can create space between the crown of the head and the tailbone. Soften your shoulders downwards to create more space in the shoulders. Release the jaw to create more space here. Take a moment to bring awareness to this idea – the sensation of space.

3. Take some time to notice the natural space between your inhalation and your exhalation. For five breaths, gently bring the navel to the spine as you breathe out.

4. Observe your thoughts for a while, seeing if you can see how they just come and go. Just let them pass without getting caught up in the thinking if you can, but it's also fine if you can't. See if you can find any small gaps between the thoughts.

5. Pick a slightly difficult but not overwhelming emotion about a situation that may be bothering you a little. Now drop your awareness into the body and just observe this as a felt sense. Where in the body do you feel this, if at all? Are the sensations strong or weak? Is there a shape or vibration? A colour? A texture or vibration? Spend a moment or two observing the physical sensation created by the emotion from the situation. If you can't feel anything, that's okay.

6. You can bring your awareness back to your Safe Resource at any time, or to the breath or the ground beneath you.

7. Bring a sense of curiosity to your physical sensations. Imagine a feeling of compassion, as if this emotion is like a small child that you are welcoming and allowing. See if you can bring a sense of kindness to how you feel.

8. Cultivate a sense of space around the physical feeling of the emotion. Feel spaciousness around and within.

9. Bring your awareness to all the people, like yourself, who have this emotion and who are perhaps in a similar situation and share your health challenges. Have a sense of gratitude for the support of others in your community, even if it's virtual. Take five breaths, visualizing light coming into the heart on every inhalation. Soften on every exhalation.

10. Take your awareness to your back. Feel space in your spine. Pause. We are now going to work through all the joints, slowly moving up from the toes, ankles, knees and hips to the fingers, feeling space in the fingers, then the wrists, elbows and shoulders. Take two breaths at each pair of joints. Spend some time with your shoulders. Now feel space in your neck.

11. Gently roll your shoulders three times very slowly. Take a moment or two to explore your shoulders and how they feel. Can you let them go a little more – even a tiny bit – are you holding on to them at all?

12. Crossing your arms over your heart, tap a few times with your fingertips on the collar bones. Then stroke down each arm with the opposite palm a few times.

13. Take your hands to your belly, then your heart, then your eyes, taking four breaths at each point. Visualize light coming into the body as the healing energy of *prana* on the inhalation.

14. Pause when you have finished and notice space between the thoughts. Observe the still point after the exhalation, before the inhalation naturally rises.

15. Come down onto the floor and place your legs on your chair so they are raised above you (unless you have heart or eye problems). You can support your head with a cushion. Use blankets for warmth, with padding under your body to keep yourself comfortable. Rest in a comfortable position, with your legs elevated.

16. Tune in to the sense of aliveness in your inner body. Observe space and peace – see if you can tune in to a sense of space and silence all around you. Even if there are noises there is also silence. Become aware of a sense of your true, authentic presence behind the thoughts. Rest, being aware of stillness, focusing on the silence between any thoughts. Drop a reflective question into the silence: 'How can I bring more space into my life?' 'How can I cultivate more peace?' Just rest here for a while, feeling safe and comfortably warm.

17. Take your hands to your heart. Breathe in peace to your heart for five slow breaths.

18. Be aware of how it feels to be calm. This is your reference point, for what it is like to feel quiet and centred. You can remember this feeling whenever you need to. It is always there for you, behind the stories that your mind spins.

19. Feel yourself surrender into the Earth. Snuggle down, resting. Believe that there is no past or future – just a sense of the sacred now, your sacred presence, and these are the same thing.

In the next two chapters we are going to explore the *chakras*, also known as our energy centres, as these are very important in terms of how we can increase our wellbeing.

KEY POINTS

✓ The Patanjali definition of yoga is to have a mind that is calm and peaceful. Yoga is also described in some scriptures as 'union'.

✓ Patanjali describes the goal of yoga as 'freedom'.

✓ Yoga is about energy. This is called *prana* in Sanskrit and is the essential vitality of all life.

✓ *Mantra* can help us to move *prana*.

✓ The breath and how we breathe is considered vital for the healthy flow of *prana*, which enters the system via *nadis*. These are channels that feed the *chakras*. Our *chakras* are centres of *prana*.

✓ *Pranayama* is an energetic practice that influences our *prana* and therefore our health. *Pranayama* means the extension of breath, and describes certain breathing techniques.

✓ *Pranayama* helps to soften and release tensions in the system. These are knots, known as *granthis* in Sanskrit.

✓ We want the breath to be slow, low and subtle. We are leading someone towards breathing more slowly, through the nose, and utilizing the diaphragm to increase health and wellbeing.

✓ *Pranayama* is considered the chief way of rejuvenating the body. It is an individual approach, and we need to be very cautious in how we proceed with this practice for those with Long Covid.

✓ The *panca maya* model, also known as the five *koshas*, describes the five interconnected dimensions that make up the human system. They are: (1) *annamaya*, the physical body; (2) *pranamaya*, our more subtle energetic system; (3) *manomaya*, the mind; (4) *vijnanamaya*, our higher mind such as wisdom and intuition; and (5) *anandamaya*, which is our bliss or spiritual true self.

✓ There are five major types of *prana* and we work with three of these for Long Covid in yoga therapy. These are:

– *Prana* itself, which is an upward-flowing energy associated with the in-breath and the chest. *Prana* can be stimulating, so we must work carefully here.

– *Apana*, a downward-flowing energy associated with the exhalation and the lower part of the body. This is considered the first energy we work with in yoga therapy, and is related to letting go and releasing.

– *Samana* around the centre of the body is about balance and harmony. It is the meeting point for *prana* and *apana*.

Chapter 6

WORKING WITH OUR ENERGY CENTRES – THE *CHAKRAS*

For our energy and health to improve it's important to have an understanding of the *chakras*. In yoga philosophy these are considered as centres for *prana*. There are many *chakras* throughout the *panca maya*, with seven major ones, but we are going to focus on the first five, as they are connected to the grounding and centring we need during a period of chronic illness such as Long Covid. These five are: *muladhara* at the base of the spine, *svadhisthana* at the sacral area, *manipura* at the navel, *anahata* at the heart region and *vishuddhi* at the region of the throat. The first two *chakras* are explained in more detail in this chapter and the next three in Chapter 7.

The *chakras* are aligned along the spine and relate to our psychological, spiritual and emotional layers as well as to how we are physically. They each have their own vibration. *Chakras* are powerful psychic centres that hold impressions and memories. It is considered that, energetically speaking, they are also where we hold trauma. In Sanskrit, the word *chakra* means a wheel or a spinning vortex of energy. All the *chakras* are connected – we can't really understand or work with one without affecting all of them. However, a *chakra* may become unbalanced, and it's possible to bring it back into balance with the appropriate yoga practice. Many of us, for example, feel ungrounded because of the busy way we live in modern society. This may cause us to be distracted without any time to process our experience. Consequently, this takes us away from our physical self and more into the head, so that we don't feel embodied. We may experience feelings of disconnection, with the mind metaphorically miles away from the present moment. Illness can add to this scenario, so the emphasis in this chapter is on balancing the lower *chakras* to help us to be more stable, present and 'in' our body.

The *chakras* can be thought of as energy stepping-stones. As we work up towards our higher centres, the vibration increases. The lower *chakras* relate to our more physical states and the higher ones are about our spiritual evolution. A *chakra* can be blocked or too open. In both cases, this can lead to physical, emotional or mental ailments related to the particular *chakra*. For example, after a bereavement, grief may open us to such overwhelming emotions that we find it difficult to manage. So, we may become overwhelmed, with little control about how we react to life. Conversely, we may shut down from uncomfortable sensations so that we detach from our current experience. Working with the heart *chakra* can help to bring either of these states back into balance. Ultimately, *chakras* are our source of wisdom, if we can learn how to listen to them. This can be challenging, but a greater awareness of what they manifest for us, both internally and externally, leads to the ability to release restrictions so that energy can flow more efficaciously. This means better health. We explore this more in what follows.

MULADHARA CHAKRA

This *chakra* is situated at the base of the spine and is also known as our root *chakra*. It is about our birth and sense of being here in this life. It is the anchor for other *chakras* and consequently is very important because it creates the foundation for how we live. This includes our sense of being grounded and stable with a feeling of trust and security in life. It is also associated with our values, how we think and our ability to let go when we need to. It is about our very sense of survival. *Muladhara* relates to the element of Earth. If this *chakra* is balanced, we have a sense of safety, a feeling of being at home, both in our bodies and the world, and a sense of knowing 'I am here'. The function of this *chakra* is nourishment. Being threatened physically (including by an illness) can unbalance *muladhara*. If there is a feeling of not wanting to exist, then the *prana* in this centre is too weak. If this *chakra* is too open and there is too much *prana*, however, because *muladhara* is associated with matter, we may grasp at material things and over-consume. This is caused by insecurity, a feeling of lack and of not having enough. This fear of being unworthy or of not really belonging is usually unconscious. However, we may think that the solution is in acquiring material goods and doing lots of shopping, because we believe this will make us more secure and help us to fit in. These are the messages of our society but this is, of course, an illusion, as security is always an inside job. Procrastination is another sign that *muladhara* needs balancing.

Every *chakra* has something called an *asura* (meaning an enemy or that which works in opposition) that can suck away at our *prana*. The *asura* of *muladhara* is fear, so we want a yoga practice that helps to overcome this. Fear has been a constant problem for many of us throughout the pandemic, partly promoted by the media and our governments, and so it is really important to do a regular grounding practice to help *muladhara* to come into balance. Restlessness, insomnia, a feeling of not being present, poor boundaries, being unfocused and difficulty in commitment are also problems that indicate that this *chakra* needs some help.

The antidote to fear is to have faith in life. So, when working with *muladhara*, we want to cultivate a sense of safety, stability and nourishment, and of really being rooted in both the body and the present moment. Practices that work on the feet and around the base of the spine are particularly good, but anything that induces a feeling of safety and being embodied is helpful. The most effective way of working with the *chakras* is to use *mantra*. The seed *mantra* for *muladhara* is 'Lam'. The 'a' when chanted is short, as in 'arm'.

LET'S PRACTISE: Grounding with the root *chakra*

1. Start by sitting in a chair. Explore how your body feels. Notice your feet on the ground. Take a moment to feel into the connection of your feet on the surface they are on, and how your hips feel against the back of the chair. Observe your physical presence in the chair and your relationship with the floor. Have a sense of the Earth or ground beneath you and the chair holding and nourishing you. Take a moment to feel into this support. With your eyes open, look around your room. Cultivate a sense of being in your space and in your body at this moment.

2. Become aware of the rhythm of your breath. Stay with this for a moment. Observe this sense of self neutrally, so there is no judgement or labelling of anything as good or bad. You are witnessing how you are with curiosity. Can you bring a sense of kindness to this observation?

3. Place your hands gently around the base of the spine. If you would like, you can chant the seed *mantra* for this *chakra*. Focusing on your sacrum area, chant 'Lam, lam, lam' three times. Alternatively, you can chant 'Om shanti'. *Shanti* means peace, and is associated with stability, nourishment and strength. This is a powerful mantra that helps to pacify fear, agitation and anxiety if chanted regularly. It's also fine to chant in English if you prefer, in which case you can chant 'Peace'.

4. Bring awareness to your feet. Observe the texture of your socks, or the floor if your feet are bare. What is the temperature under your feet? Is the floor soft or hard? Are there any vibrations or sensations? Take a moment to observe and explore this. Now spread your toes and have a sense of your feet softening and widening on the floor. Feel the two surfaces – the soles of the feet and the floor.

5. Cultivate a sense of gratitude for the support of the Earth below you, if you can. Breathe in, visualizing inhaling up through your feet, up your body, into your heart centre. Breathe down and out through the feet, allowing the Earth to take away anything negative on the exhalation. Visualize the in-breath nourishing you as the Earth brings you stability.

6. Come down to a comfortable lying position with the knees bent and some support under your head. Take a moment to feel the safety of the Earth holding you. Allow your body to soften into your support. You can remain sitting if you prefer.

7. If you are lying on your back, you are going to practise gentle twisting. Otherwise, visualize the next movements. Take your arms out to the sides like a cross, slightly

below shoulder level. Palms can be down or up, whatever is comfortable. Knees are bent and legs hip width apart, heels in line with your buttocks. Inhale. Exhaling, take the knees slowly towards the right, with the movement following the breath. Pause for two breaths. On each exhalation, allow your knees to soften down towards the floor.

8. Roll your head to look over your left shoulder, keeping both shoulders aligned on the floor. Now inhale and centre the knees and the head. Exhaling, take your knees towards the left, rolling your head towards the right. Again, stay for two breaths, allowing the knees to soften towards the floor on the out-breath. Repeat up to twice more on each side, working slowly and mindfully with the breath. Pause as you centre yourself. Gently bring both knees over your belly and rock from side to side.

9. Take some time, exploring the rocking sensation. Feel the sensation of the floor under your lower back. You can make small movements or larger ones. Now rest, being aware of the floor supporting you and your physical connection with your support.

10. Continue to relax in a position that is comfortable for you. Observe how you are feeling – emotionally, energetically, mentally and physically. Can you be with everything as it is? Even pain and fatigue – can you just allow everything to be as it is, observing it neutrally?

11. If you are on your back, bend your knees and remove anything from under your head. Your feet are hip width apart and your hands are palms face down beside your hips.

12. Bring your awareness into your feet. Gently lift one foot and then the other, really paying attention to the sensations in your feet. Stamp your feet up and down gently on the floor a few times. Now spread your toes.

13. Bring awareness to your hands, feeling the texture of your surface under the palms. Spread your fingers.

14. Become aware of the base of your spine. How is your lower back feeling? If comfortable, gently lift your hips to raise up onto your shoulders as you inhale, keeping your knees stable and your chin tucked into your chest, so you are keeping the length in the back of the neck. Gently push your feet and hands into the floor as you lift your hips. As you exhale, slowly, and in time with the breath, come down. Rest or repeat the movement up to three more times, depending on your energy levels. Keep your awareness in your feet and base of your spine as you lift and come down. Be aware of the support of the Earth under you, always there for you.

15. Rest for a few minutes. When you are ready, roll to one side. Pause, especially if you have PoTS. When you are ready, come back to sitting on a chair with your feet on the floor. If they won't reach the floor, place a cushion or block there. Have your back well supported, maybe with cushions.

16. Observe your posture. Feel your sit bones against the seat of the chair, feet are firmly on the floor, hip width apart. Sit as if your spine is rising up from your base like a spring. Open your ribs and allow the top of your chest to float up. Roll your shoulders once or twice, then draw the shoulders gently together and relax them down. Lift your chin as if you were nodding upwards, then tuck the chin into the top of your chest so that the back of the neck is lengthened. Feel the connection with the top of the head and the base of the spine, and visualize space opening between these two points.

17. Become aware of the breath. Focus for up to 10 breaths on a long, smooth exhalation. If you can, breathe through your nose, but it's also fine if you can't.

18. Bring awareness back to your feet. Spend a moment or two feeling into the connection of your feet on the floor or cushion. Bring awareness to your bottom on the chair. Feel yourself supported by the chair and observe any sensation for a moment or two. Is there any tingling? Vibration? Now bring your awareness to the base of the spine. Feel your lower back against your support. Pause, resting your awareness here for a few moments.

19. Decide which one of these three points to focus on. Your feet, or your bottom, or the base of your spine. Choose one. Bring your full attention to the point you have chosen. Observe the temperature, texture, sensations, vibrations and anything else about the point you are focused on. Try to keep your awareness there. If the mind wanders, gently bring it back. Stay with your focus for around 3 minutes. On every exhalation, feel that you are letting go through your point of attention, into the ground.

20. Gently, widen your awareness to incorporate the whole of the physical body. Starting at the feet, slowly scan your body up to the crown of the head. Pause. Inhale up through the base of the spine to the crown of the head for five slow, mindful breaths. On the exhalation, feel the breath moving out down the feet and into the Earth. Feel that the breath is nourishing you. Be aware of your feet planted on the Earth, with the ground supporting you. Take several breaths like this before you then come back to normal breathing. Allow yourself to become still, just observing how you are. Body, mind and emotions, just allowing everything to be as it is.

21. With your fingers, gently massage around the jaw, then the shoulders and down the arms. Then relax the jaw and eyes.

22. Take your hands and place them on your heart, bringing your awareness here. Softly breathe in a sense of light into the heart for five breaths. If you would like, you can chant 'Lam, lam' again a few times, or 'Om shanti' or 'Peace, peace'.

23. Sit quietly, allowing whatever arises to be there without trying to change anything. Focus on the support you feel beneath you, and the sensation of being in your body.

SVADHISTHANA CHAKRA

This *chakra* is about movement, flow and creativity. *Svadhisthana* relates to the area around the pelvis, and is represented by the element of Water. It is considered to be our source of power. It is also about what we manifest in life and how we can innovate something into being. If we can visualize ideas as love, light, creativity, kindness and compassion as we create something material, then we can nurture and grow this into many forms (such as is expressed by art, cooking, childrearing, music, movement, or just by how we live). This beauty then spreads outwards to everyone in the world. When *svadhisthana* is in balance, we can nurture ourselves as well as others and are able to give and receive within relationships. This means we are comfortable within sexual intimacy. Because this *chakra* is about creation, we can have fun and can explore both our creativity and also our sexuality with confidence.

If *prana* is weak in this *chakra*, we may become rigid on any dimension of the *panca maya*. This means we will fear any kind of change, so our body, mind or emotions may appear as inflexible. This can manifest as lack of enjoyment for life and an inability to appreciate music, food or any sensual pleasure. Not enough *prana* in *svadhisthana* may also show up as social anxiety. Conversely, if there is too much *prana*, this can manifest as mood swings or an addiction to pleasure and drama. Poor boundaries within relationships and emotional dependence on others is also a sign of lack of harmony at this centre.

The sacral *chakra* is about balancing our masculine and feminine energies, which also represent a sense of healthy contraction and expansion in life. The breath is reflected in this – the inhale is expansive whereas the exhalation contracts, and there should be a coherent balance of these two. When *svadhisthana* is healthy, there is balance, we enjoy life and our connection to others, and we can also function individually at our full creative potential.

The enemy (*asura*) of this *chakra* is guilt. This may be for many reasons, even going back to childhood. There may also be a feeling of guilt associated with having Long Covid because of not being well enough to 'do' or 'contribute', or of being seen as lazy. We can help to counteract this with an appropriate yoga practice together with some self-inquiry. The seed *mantra* for *svadhisthana* is 'Vam'.

LET'S PRACTISE: Playing creatively with the sacral *chakra*

This practice encompasses eye movements that are particularly powerful because the vagus nerve and eye movements are interconnected. Moving the eyes creates a connection to the muscles that sit at the base of the skull. As the eyes change position, this creates subtle movements that help to release tight muscles in the neck. This, in turn, can reduce tension around the first and second cervical vertebrae, helping to relieve neck and eye pain and headaches. This also takes us out of the fixed eye focus created by the stress response. We have included these eye movements here, because as well as being extremely beneficial, they can also be playful.

1. Sit comfortably upright in a chair, or lie on your front or back. Take a moment or two to come into the body, noticing how everything is – mind, body, energy, emotions. Ask yourself these questions: 'How am I?' and 'What do I need?' Take a moment to observe your state of being without judgement, bringing a sense of compassion to how you are in this moment. See if you can develop a quality of non-resistance, accepting everything as it is. Observe your whole state of being with kindness.

2. Take your hands to your pelvic area. If you would rather not do this, you can visualize the area below the belly and the mid-spine. If you would like, chant the seed *mantra* 'Vam, vam, vam' a few times. As an alternative, you may like to hum the breath out between closed lips for up to five slow breaths.

3. Take your arms out to the sides and wave them about slowly and gently, playing with the sensation of movement. Imagine that you are waving them through water. Just try this for a few seconds so that you are not tiring yourself. Be aware of how your arms and hands feel in space/water, and also how your shoulders are with this movement.

4. Now roll your shoulders slowly 3–5 times.

5. Staying in contact with the chair or surface you are on, make a large circle from your pelvic area, circling your body first one way and then the other. Explore this movement a few times. Then rock slowly from side to side, experimenting and playing with the motion.

6. Become aware of the breath and allow it to be as it is. After a few minutes, and if it's comfortable, begin to slow the breath down. Have one hand on the belly and one on the heart. Breathe in softly and gently to the hand on the belly. Breathe in through the nose – if comfortable. If you feel anxious at any time about following the breath, bring your awareness to the softness of the hands or to your Safe Resource. Using balanced (*samana*) breathing, take up to 10 breaths with an even inhale and exhale.

7. If you are sitting, come down to lying comfortably. Arms are slightly away from the body with the palms turned up or down, or rest them on your belly. Knees are bent. Support your head with some padding. Observe the rise and fall of the belly in time with the breath for a moment or two, using your Safe Resource at any time you need.

8. Slowly roll your head from side to side. Observe how the neck is and the weight of the head. Centre the head. Focus on releasing and relaxing the body into your support with every exhalation. Become aware of your back. Observe where your back is touching your support (or front/side if you are not on your back) and also notice where there are spaces.

9. Become aware of your hands and arms. As you breathe in, inhale an orange light up your right arm into the pelvis, visualizing that you are bringing energy into *svadhisthana chakra* on this in-breath. On the exhalation, breathe down your left

arm, letting the breath take away anything you don't want. Imagine the in-breath as a sense of receiving power from the Earth and the exhalation as a sense of giving back to the Earth. Feel the balance of the breath – the inhalation and the exhalation. If comfortable, count to four slowly as you inhale, and four as you exhale. If that's too much, alter your counting. If you don't like focusing on the breath, just visualize the colours.

10. If on your back, open your eyes and bend your knees. Visualize a clock face around your pelvis, with 6 o'clock at the bottom and 12 o'clock at the top towards the belly button; 3 o'clock is at the left side of the pelvis and 9 o'clock at the right side. You are going to circle around your pelvis, and as you do so, let your eyes also slowly circle in time with the knees, by gazing at each point of an imagined clock face.

11. Begin to circle the pelvis around the clock face, allowing the knees to relax as you do so. Starting at 12, slightly tilt your pelvis as your lower back connects with the floor. Gaze down towards the imagined 12 o'clock point, near your belly button. Slowly roll around so your knees flop slightly to the left towards 3 o'clock, taking your gaze down towards the left. Next roll to 6, so the pelvis is tilted away from you and you are now gazing towards the bottom of the pelvis. Roll the pelvis towards the right side at 9 o'clock, letting the knees come to the right with the eyes looking down and right. Come back to 12 o'clock with the eyes and the pelvis. Observe how you are also circling around the base of your spine. How does that feel? Be curious and playful if you can. Make a few more slow circles of your pelvis and eyes clockwise, then repeat the other way, going anti-clockwise. Pause when you have finished. Focus on the area around your pelvis and lower back. Rest with your eyes closed if you would like, pelvis now in a neutral position, with the knees still bent, feet hip width apart.

12. A gentle variation of this is to lie on your back with knees bent and arms out to the side. Eyes are open, but feel free to blink. Start by gazing at the ceiling for five breaths. Then, keeping the face still and soft, roll the eyes to gaze down towards your left thumb (don't worry if you can't actually see it). Take five breaths, looking down towards the thumb. Next, return your gaze back to the centre looking at the ceiling for five breaths. Now, keeping the jaw and face still and soft, roll the eyes to look down towards the right thumb and hold the gaze there for five breaths. Centre the gaze back to the ceiling for five more breaths. Then close your eyes and relax.

13. Draw your knees in towards your belly, then rock slowly from side to side.

14. Observe the effects of the practice so far. Can you become aware of the still point after the exhalation? Can you bring a sense of kindness to how your whole being is right in this moment?

15. Gently lift the knees and bring them together. Roll to one side. Rest and slowly move into a Cat position with your hands under the shoulders and knees under the hips, using support under the knees if needed. You can also do this movement from a chair. If kneeling, spread your fingers, being aware of the palms of the hands connecting with the floor.

16. Observe the space between the crown of the head and your tailbone, and visualize space in the spine between these two points. Now become aware of your pelvis.

17. Slowly circle your pelvis one way three or four times, then the other way. Make the movement playful and creative. You can bring the arms and legs in if you like – waving one arm in the air or one leg, then swapping limbs.

18. Come back to the centre. Pause. Now, inhale and lift the heart, then exhale and round the spine slightly, bringing the navel to the spine on the out-breath. Flow with this movement for a few breaths, with the movement following the breath.

19. Lie on your front, or if you are unable to, visualize the next movements. Either bend the elbows and rest your forehead on the backs of the hands or roll your head to one side and have the arms beside you, palms up. If your neck becomes tired, roll the head to the other side.

20. Become aware of the breath in the belly. As you inhale, feel the slight pressure of the belly against the floor. Feel this pressure release on the exhalation and gently draw your navel to your spine. Observe for a few breaths.

21. Bend your knees, raising the soles of the feet toward the ceiling. Sway the legs gently from side to side.

22. Rest on the front or back, just observing how everything is.

KEY POINTS

✓ A *chakra* is a wheel or a spinning vortex of energy.

✓ The *chakras* are centres for *prana*. They can be too open, with too much *prana*, or too closed. Through an appropriate yoga practice we can bring them into balance.

✓ Our *chakras* are aligned along the spine and relate to our psychological, spiritual and emotional layers as well as to how we are physically.

✓ We can think of the *chakras* as energy stepping-stones. As we work upwards, the vibration increases. The lower *chakras* relate to our physical states and the higher ones to our spiritual evolution.

✓ For Long Covid, we are concerned with the first five *chakras*.

✓ Every *chakra* has an individual seed *mantra*. Chanting this can help with the health of each *chakra* over time.

✓ *Muladhara*, also known as the root *chakra*, is at the base of the spine. It is about our sense of being here in this life and in our body.

✓ It is also about our sense of being grounded and having faith in life.

✓ *Muladhara* relates to the element of Earth, and its function is nourishment.

✓ If this *chakra* is balanced, we have a feeling of being at home in our body.

✓ Fear, restlessness, anxiety, insomnia and a feeling of not being in the body indicate that *prana* is low in this *chakra*.

✓ Embodiment, grounding and somatic practices can help to balance *muladhara chakra*.

✓ *Svadhisthana*, or our sacral *chakra*, is around the pelvic area. It is about movement, flow and creativity.

✓ This *chakra* is our source of power. It is about giving and receiving, which is reflected in our relationships, including sexual intimacy. It is our source of creation.

✓ *Svadhisthana* is about balancing our masculine and feminine energies. This is reflected by the inhalation and exhalation as we balance expansion and contraction.

✓ The element of *svadhisthana* is Water.

Chapter 7

RAISING ENERGY – THE *CHAKRAS*

MANIPURA CHAKRA

Manipura chakra (known as *manipuraka* in some traditions) is our sun centre and is associated with the qualities of digestion and transformation. *Manipura* combines matter and movement, and is about our sense of will. It is represented by the element of Fire. Transformation can happen on all levels – for example, the digestion and transformation of food into energy, but also digestion and transformation of our experiences and emotions when they are processed healthily. This helps us to learn and grow. *Manipura* is an important *chakra* for vitality because it is associated with motivation, ego, autonomy and will power. These need to be in balance, so that we can function as a unique human being with a positive sense of self. If *muladhara* is 'I am', *manipura* is 'I am here' – it's about being here in the world, rather than just in the body. Although our spiritual progress in yoga is ultimately about union, we also need a healthy sense of self as an individual, so that we can separate our own intentions and experiences from those of others. Then we understand that we are acting from what is right for us, rather than being disempowered and manipulated into living in ways that suit only external authority and the desire of others. When this *chakra* is balanced, we have a good sense of who we are internally and how we relate to the world externally.

This centre can easily become imbalanced by external circumstances, especially by those who hold power and who may encourage us into destructive behaviours. Hyperactivity, being over-ambitious or driven to the point of burnout are signs that *prana* may be too strong here. Power can be destructive and intoxicating, so energy ends up dissipating itself. Over-consumption of food, news, experiences or information, for example, can lead to overwhelm, as we rush from one thing to another, leaving no time to digest anything. Consequently, we have no space for positive transformation to happen. At the global level, we see the desire for power destroying the world and its inhabitants. We might call this a gross imbalance of *manipura chakra*.

If *prana* is too weak at this centre, there may be lack of will power with no self-discipline, and even a victim mentality. Someone with poor boundaries, who always puts others before themselves without taking enough time to focus on self-worth or care, will benefit by working with *manipura*. Certainly, our personal experience is that those who lack self-compassion can lose themselves in the desires and needs of others, and this can eventually lead to illness. Depression, exhaustion, repressed emotions, digestive disorders such as IBS and being collapsed around the middle are other indications that *prana* is weak in *manipura*. From the yogic point of view, chronic fatigue is thought to be an imbalance here. At the physical level (*annamaya*), this *chakra* relates to the sides of the body, the ribs, the centre of the spine, the digestion and also the diaphragm, which we know is vital for healthy breathing. Any restriction in this area will have a negative impact on both health and energy.

When this *chakra* is in balance, we see someone who is confident and reliable with a warm personality and healthy sense of self. With *manipura* in harmony, we are naturally proactive, with the discipline to complete tasks but also an understanding of limits and when to stop.

The enemy (*asura*) of this *chakra* is shame. This happens if we are dominated by others – in other words, when our vulnerability and our right to act as we wish is disrespected, or when something is forced upon us. Many in our society refuse to acknowledge illnesses such as ME/CFS and Long Covid, so shame may be a part of the lived experience of having an illness that is belittled, questioned or even denied. The seed *mantra* of *manipura* is 'Ram'.

LET'S PRACTISE: *Manipura* – sun centring

1. Sit comfortably, upright either on the floor or in a chair. Take the hands and place them on the belly.

2. Chant the seed *mantra* if you would like: 'Ram, ram, ram.' The ' r' should be rolled like a motorcycle, and is short. Chant for three out breaths, with confidence. As always, chanting is optional.

3. Close your eyes and visualize golden light at the belly. On the inhalation visualize the light glowing brightly. Exhale slowly, allowing the out-breath to be longer than the in-breath. Repeat 3–5 times slowly.

4. Come down to lying comfortably on your back with the knees bent, feet hip width apart. Resting your hands on the belly, visualize light coming into the belly as you inhale. On the exhalation, visualize this light as healing *prana*, sending energy to wherever you need it. As always, if you are not comfortable on your back, remain seated or lie on your front if you prefer. Pause and observe for a few breaths.

5. Now lie in the shape of an X with legs and arms wide apart. The knees can remain bent if you have any pain or discomfort in the back. The arms can come lower down to shoulder level if your shoulders are tight.

6. Visualize a wheel of gentle sunlight at the navel. As you breathe in, visualize taking in light to the navel, watching it glow brighter. Exhale, sending the light to the whole body, seeing it travelling up the arms and down the legs. Take a few breaths like this.

7. Relax, bringing the legs further together, and take the arms to beside the hips, slightly away from the body, with the palms turned up. Spend a moment or two observing how you feel – mind, body, emotions and energy. Just tune in to the 'weather pattern' of how you are. Try to do this without judging anything. See if you can observe yourself neutrally or, even better, with kindness.

8. Draw the knees over the belly, taking one knee over and then the other. Hold around or under the knees. Following the breath, inhale and let the arms straighten as you float the knees away from you. Exhale and gently draw the knees in towards you. Repeat 3–5 times. If you would like, you can combine this movement with the chant. As you gently bring the knees into the belly, on the out-breath chant 'Ram, ram, ram'. Alternatively, you can chant 'Light, light, light'.

9. Relax with the knees softly into the belly and observe your whole self neutrally. See if you can bring a sense of spaciousness to your state of being – just as it is in this moment. Allow everything to be as it is. Observe the still point after the exhalation. Stay for a few breaths.

10. We are going to move into Bridge posture. In the practice for *muladhara chakra*, we focused on the feet and base of the spine. For *manipura*, we will bring awareness to the belly, visualizing it filling with light as the navel lifts towards the ceiling.

11. Have the feet hip width apart, heels in line with the buttocks. Arms are beside the body with the palms down. Take away any support from under your head and lengthen your neck by tucking the chin into the chest.

12. Inhale, visualizing light in the belly as you lift your hips to come up onto your shoulders. Gently press on the hands and feet to stabilize your body and to keep the knees from drifting apart. Keep the back of the neck long. Stay for two breaths, lifting the light-filled belly up higher on each inhalation. Then come back down on the next exhale. You can repeat once or twice or just rest down, depending on energy levels. As always, listen to your body and be kind to yourself. If you need to rest, then rest.

13. Relax with your legs on a chair and a cushion under your head. Observe your breathing, focusing on a slow, smooth exhalation. Hum the breath out with closed lips for five slow breaths, or chant 'Ram, ram, ram'. Feel your body becoming softer with every out-breath. You might like to visualize gentle fire in your belly, burning everything you want to let go of as you relax. Stay here, resting for a while.

14. Roll to the side to come out of the inversion and stay there resting. When you are ready, spiral up to sitting to carry on with your day.

ANAHATA CHAKRA

Anahata chakra at the heart region is our centre of pure altruistic love and connection. When this *chakra* is in balance, all our actions are taken with compassion and authenticity for self and for others. Often called the 'site of that which cannot be destroyed', this *chakra* is known as our centre of light and is the home of our true radiant being. The heart centre is the gateway from the lower, more Earth-bound *chakras* to the higher spiritual ones and there needs to be a balance between them, so that we are neither too materialistic and Earth-bound, nor too floaty and ethereal.

The heart *chakra* is associated with the divine, and it is said that the individual spirit resides here. When we are living from our hearts as opposed to our heads, we act from a sense of truth and wisdom. To live authentically takes much courage, as it may involve bypassing the fear of the ego that wants something different. It may even mean going against the narrative of the wider community. Yet if we are to fully heal from illness, the journey to the heart means cultivating courage to live in a way that honours our personal truth and allows us to be vulnerable when necessary, so we can drop our *kavacam*. (Remember this word from Chapter 2 – it means our protective veil or false self.) This means our thoughts, words and deeds are always in alignment, and we are not thinking or saying one thing, then acting in a different way. In the Vedic tradition, love is not just about the relationship that we have with others, but also about the relationship we have with ourselves, because this helps us to have a genuine heartfelt connection to those we come into contact with.

The element of this *chakra* is Wind and its purpose is balance. We see this best with our breath which, through *pranayama*, can help to balance all of the *chakras*, including the heart centre. It is said that when we are in love, there is a special breath, with the inhalation bringing us inspiration and vitality. The enemy (*asura*) of the heart centre is grief, especially if this is repressed. Betrayal and loss can also cause *prana* in this centre to weaken, as can living in a cold, loveless environment. This may manifest in someone as poor boundaries, anti-social behaviour or intolerance and judgement of self as well as of others. Someone with low *prana* here can then be easily manipulated by others, because of this disconnection and lack of self-compassion. A person who is isolated and lonely with a fear of intimacy is also likely to have low *prana* at the heart. Death, divorce and separation are all challenges to this *chakra*. At the physical level (*annamaya*), lack of *prana* may cause us to hunch over to protect the heart, restricting the chest, lungs, diaphragm and, of course, the breath. A sunken chest or any shoulder problems also indicates an imbalance at *anahata*.

Conversely, if there is too much *prana*, we may become clingy, co-dependent and live our lives through others. Burnout from over-giving, depression or heart and breathing difficulties are all key signs that *prana* in the heart needs to be balanced. With the advent of Covid, which affects the heart and lungs, we have contemplated that globally this was a sign that we all need to live more from the heart and less from the head. In other words, we should live as truthfully as possible, rather than from just our over-analytical minds.

When the heart *chakra* is in harmony, we feel safe, we are in tune with ourselves and others, and we are able to listen to and act from a sense of our authentic intuition, unclouded by the antics of a busy mind. For this, we need to take time in silence or meditation every day. We can work with this *chakra* physically by gently encouraging the heart centre to lift and expand. When we live from a place of sincerity, we are naturally compassionate and loving to ourselves as well as to others. We have better immunity and a sense of peace and calm, even in times of difficulty and change. This *chakra* helps us to discriminate between what is right and wrong because we are listening to our true inner voice – the light in the heart that always guides us with wisdom. The seed *mantra* for this *chakra* is 'Yam'.

LET'S PRACTISE: *Anahata* – opening the heart

1. Sit comfortably upright, preferably in a chair. Explore the sensation of your feet against the floor (using a cushion or block under your feet if necessary). Take a moment to settle. Become curious about how you feel – emotionally, energetically, mentally and physically. How is your breath? Try not to judge, just observe.

2. Gently roll your shoulders a few times, first lifting them, then drawing the shoulder blades together before releasing the shoulders down. Then lift your sternum (top of the chest) gently without strain, so that your lower ribs naturally open.

3. Place your hands at your heart – either with palms pressed together in prayer *mudra* or hands one on top of the other. Drop your awareness into your heart. Take a moment to be still. Does your heart have a message for you? Pause, allowing everything to be. Listen. It's fine if there is no message – just feel the physical sensation around the heart.

4. As always, chanting is optional. If you would like, chant 'Om yam, yam, yam' three times or 'Love, love, love' if you prefer. Chant this to your heart with a sense of genuine love if you can. If love is too difficult to access, chant with a sense of kindness. It's also fine to hum on the out-breath or to remain silent.

5. Keep the left hand on the heart and take the right hand to the belly. If it's comfortable, breathe softly into the belly, feeling the hand move slightly. The hand on the heart is pacifying the chest area. If you are able to, breathe through your nose. Take up to 10 breaths, but only if this is comfortable. Think of the breath being slow and low.

6. Take both hands back to the heart. Start with the palms together, then soften them to make space between the palms. This is *anjali mudra*.

7. Inhaling, open your arms wide. Exhaling and crossing the arms over, give yourself a hug. Take up to five slow, mindful breaths like this. Really enjoy the hug and sense of touch.

8. Stroke slowly down the arms with the opposite hands a few times.

9. We are going to practise seated Cat. Inhale and lift your heart, keeping your chin slightly in so that the back of the neck is long. Exhale, taking the navel to the spine and round the spine slightly, dropping the head down. Take five breaths like this, then come back to a neutral seated position with neck, head and spine in line. Pause for a few breaths.

10. Focus on breathing a sense of light into the heart on every inhalation, and directing this light to wherever you need some healing on the exhalation. Repeat 3–5 times.

11. Come to lie on your front, if you would like. Remember, everything is always a choice. Either rest your forehead on the back of your hands, one hand on top of the other, or take your head to one side with the arms beside the body, palms up. Roll your head to the other side if your neck feels stiff. Rest here for a few minutes. It's fine to remain sitting if this is more comfortable, in which case you can visualize the next sequence.

12. Bring your forehead to the centre. Bend your elbows and align them with your chest. Inhale, and lift up the heart centre, coming up onto your elbows. Keep a sense of release between the shoulder blades. Keep your lower navel on the ground.

13. Continue to breathe, sensing the feeling of your elbows rooting down into the floor. If you can, lift the front body slightly more. Next, direct the elbows towards your waist, opening the heart centre. Let the head rise naturally in line with the upper back, keeping the navel connected with the floor. Look forward, keeping the chin in and lengthening the back of the neck. Draw the shoulder blades together as you lift your heart *chakra*. Move between relaxing down back to the floor on the exhale and then lifting and opening the heart space to rise up slightly on the inhale. Lift and lower a few times. Rest down whenever you need.

14. Rest in any way which feels right, maybe coming onto your back or staying on your front. Take a moment to notice the effect of the practice on all levels of your being. Observe for a few slow breaths.

15. Visualize a circle of loved ones surrounding you. These may be friends, relatives, teachers or inspirational figures. Maybe you have pets who can join you too. Take a moment or two to feel this circle of loved ones around you.

16. Focus on the feeling of your circle of care sending love to you. All these beings who mean something to you are sending you their good wishes and love. Bathe in the feeling of their compassionate unconditional love. Visualize that you are breathing this in through your heart, absorbing love into your whole being. Inhale and exhale through the heart.

17. You may like to contemplate that this love comes from you and is not something that is separate or external. Still breathing from the heart, direct this love to yourself, from yourself.

VISHUDDHI CHAKRA

Do you always say what you mean? Do you sometimes hide behind a veil of polite people pleasing? If our heart *chakra* is about cultivating unconditional love and authenticity, *vishuddhi*, at the throat area, is about how we express our deepest truth. *Vishuddhi chakra* is associated with the element of Space. We need space for heart-to-heart connection and for the ability to listen and understand. If we want to express something but feel that we can't, then we literally 'swallow' our feelings and this becomes a toxic knot (*granthi*), causing us stress and tension, and eventually illness.

There is a principle in yoga that words and sound can change matter. Vedic philosophy suggests that, for health, we should elevate and purify our voice with *mantra*. Ultimately this raises our vibration so that we can express our authenticity. Chanting, prayer and the appropriate use of the voice are therefore very important for this *chakra*, as is the freedom to communicate our personal truth. This means conveying what the heart feels, so that there is a cohesion of mind, feeling, action and words. Then we are aligned with life, which consequently becomes smoother and less chaotic. Living and expressing truth with kindness has the power to take us out of our suffering. Our conditioned patterns, however, may veil our authentic self, and this may cause us problems as we repeatedly act without awareness. For example, maybe we say what we think others want to hear rather than what we really mean and so we end up feeling resentful, stressed and misunderstood. This often shows up in relationships. Having the courage to be truthful, however, breaks this pattern. Working with *vishuddhi* means we communicate everything with gentle, tactful but appropriate authority. Silence and the ability to apply deep conscious listening to others is also associated with the balance of this *chakra*, as is the health of the throat, neck and shoulders.

The enemy (*asura*) of this *chakra* is being lied to, being given mixed messages and any form of verbal abuse such as being yelled at or being subject to excessive criticism. Keeping secrets will also unbalance this centre. Yet again, we might consider what has gone on in our society during the pandemic and beyond, with censorship and control. At challenging times such as we are living through now, it becomes even more important that we speak with verity, whatever the cost. Truth, asserted from the heart, is very different from opinion or the kind of binary communication that so often is voiced, all too often aggressively, in the world.

When *prana* is low in this centre we may fear speaking out. The voice may be weak, with no ability to project. There may be a problem with reporting feelings or a constriction of expression. Conversely, if *prana* is too strong, there may be over-talking, poor listening skills, or verbal manipulation and aggression. It can be difficult to follow the conversation of someone with an unbalanced throat *chakra*, as the speech jumps about. When this *chakra* is balanced, however, the voice is resonant and sweet. There is no ambiguity but coherent, dignified, kind communication. The seed *mantra* for this *chakra* is 'Ham'.

LET'S PRACTISE: *Vishuddhi* – expressing our truth

1. Come to a comfortable sitting position. Take a moment or two to notice your posture. Feel the space between the crown of the head and the tailbone. Nod the head up, then down, and lengthen the back of the neck, tucking the chin in slightly to the top of the chest.

2. Gently roll your shoulders two or three times, drawing the shoulder blades together and then releasing them down, away from the ears.

3. Breathe in. As you exhale, take your left ear towards your left shoulder. Inhale and centre your head. Exhale and take your right ear towards your right shoulder. Inhale and centre the head. Repeat twice more to each side. Keep the shoulders relaxed.

4. Take a moment or two just to sit quietly, noticing how you are in this moment. Soften the area around the throat. How do you feel? How is the mind? Can you observe your whole state of being without judgement?

5. Become aware of your breath, if this is okay for you. See if you can breathe lightly through your nose, with the idea of breathing slow and low, so that you are engaging your diaphragm. To help with this, you might like to take the navel to the spine gently on the exhalation. If this is not yet possible, breathe in a way that feels right for you.

6. Take your hands either side of your lower rib cage so your thumbs point around your back and your fingers curl around the ribs. As you inhale, feel the ribs gently flare outward. As you exhale, very gently squeeze the ribs towards each other. Take 3–5 breaths like this, if this feels all right.

7. Drop your hands to your knees. See if you can observe the gentle pause after the exhalation before the inhalation naturally starts. The inhale is free. Just focus on the sense of this natural space after the out-breath.

8. If you would like to chant, gently touch your fingertips around your throat. Chant 'Om, ham, ham, ham' three times. If you would prefer, you can hum the breath out instead, or remain silent.

9. Pause, feeling the effects and the silence created by the *mantra*.

10. Gently take your hands and place them either side of your face, so you are holding your face with a sense of compassion. Take three gentle and mindful breaths here.

11. Take your left palm onto your forehead and your right palm around the base of the head. Cradling your head with kindness, take three gentle breaths.

12. Keep one hand on your forehead and take one hand to your heart. Take three more slow and mindful breaths.

13. Drop the hand on the forehead onto the belly. Take three gentle mindful breaths.

14. Sit quietly on your chair and just observe. Then when you are ready, chant 'Om, ham, ham, ham' or hum, if you prefer, up to three more times on the exhale.

15. Sit quietly for a few minutes just enjoying the feeling of space and quietness.

There are two more major *chakras* that are associated with our spiritual progress. These are *ajna* at the eyebrow centre, sometimes known as the third eye, and *sahasrara* at the crown of the head. However, in this book we have just covered the *chakras* we think are the most important for helping those with Long Covid and fatigue in their recovery journey.

KEY POINTS

✓ *Manipura chakra*, at our navel centre, is known as our sun centre. It is associated with digestion and transformation.

✓ The element of this *chakra* is Fire. It is also concerned with motivation, autonomy and will power.

✓ *Manipura* is also about having a healthy sense of self in our relationship to the world.

✓ When this *chakra* is in balance, we are confident and reliable.

✓ *Anahata chakra* at the heart centre is the place of pure, altruistic love and connection. It is about compassion and authenticity, both for self and for others.

✓ The element of the heart *chakra* is Wind and the purpose is balance.

✓ *Anahata* is also known as the site of 'that which cannot be destroyed' and our centre of light. It is where the individual spirit resides.

✓ *Anahata* is the gateway of our lower, more Earth-bound *chakras* to our higher spiritual ones.

✓ When we come from the heart, our thoughts, words and deeds are in alignment, and we can live our personal truth.

✓ To balance this *chakra*, we should take time in silence every day. We can also work with chest-opening postures that help to open the heart, such as Cobra and Sphinx.

✓ *Vishuddhi* is the throat *chakra*. It is located around the throat, neck and shoulders.

✓ The element of this *chakra* is Space.

✓ *Vishuddhi* is about authentic expression and the ability to listen deeply to others.

✓ There is a principle in yoga that words and sound can change matter. Therefore, for our health, we should purify this *chakra* with *mantra*, prayer, chanting and the appropriate use of the voice. This helps to raise our vibration.

✓ Balancing *vishuddhi* helps us to express our truth with kindness, communicating what the heart feels rather than what our ego or conditioning tells us to say.

✓ Freedom of expression is important for our health so that we are not swallowing our words and we can say what we really mean.

✓ When this *chakra* is in balance, we communicate to others with tactful, appropriate and gentle authority.

✓ The voice of someone with the throat *chakra* in balance is resonant and sweet, with clarity and coherence.

Chapter 8

RESTING AND RELAXATION FOR RECOVERY

THE IMPORTANCE OF REST FOR RECOVERY

Deep rest is your superpower when it comes to healing. The UK (National Health Service, NHS) and US (Centers for Disease Control and Prevention, CDC) recommendations for recovery from Covid-19 propose that people should rest as much as possible during the active infection to decrease the risk of Long Covid, and also to manage the condition (Drew 2023). However, they remain vague as to *how* we should rest. Claudia Hammond, Professor of Psychology, defines rest as an activity that is 'restorative, intentional, relaxing' (Hammond and Lewis 2016). Individual perception of what rest is varies widely. However, when it comes to recovery from a chronic illness such as Long Covid, we know that the biggest factor in healing is proper breathing, serious convalescence and regular periods of quiet relaxation.

Deep rest (and in our opinion, this means not even listening to a podcast, scrolling social media or watching TV) allows the nervous system to restore, so that the body can get on with the repair it needs. In terms of Ayurveda (often called the sister science of yoga), resting increases *kapha*, the element that can help to boost immunity. So judicious resting (not too much, but definitely not too little) is vital for healing. Sadly, many of us find taking rest difficult, either because patterns of perfectionism, pleasing and overdoing things puts us into a habitual chronic stress response and we find it difficult to come out of that kind of activation, or because our busy lifestyles mean we don't prioritize the importance of taking time out to let our nervous system replenish. Furthermore, resting can be challenging because we may initially feel more achy and tired as the 'rest and digest' branch of the PNS takes time with its healing. But stopping regularly to take deep rest is a vital habit (a new *samskara*) to acquire if we are to get better and address chronic nervous system dysregulation.

We asked people with Long Covid and ME/CFS how easy they found it to rest. Some of the comments included:

My relationship with rest changes regularly and is hugely impacted by (and can also tell me a lot about) where I'm at with trauma processing at any moment. This additional layer makes fatigue recovery particularly challenging at times.

During my worst times my body couldn't relax: too much adrenaline, cortisol and overall hypervigilance. Slowly, slowly understanding what was going on physically and mentally really helped me to persevere. I have struggled to relax at times and still find I put the care of others before self-care. But the family knows that afternoons are for me to rest and they respect that. Slow deep breathing helps.

Yes, I absolutely find it difficult to rest! It's worse when I've done too much that day and need to rest more than ever.

I remember being told by a fatigue specialist that 'sleep doesn't relieve fatigue, rest does'. This helped me relax my attitude around sleep, so I'm less anxious about bad nights. I have since prioritized daily 'rest' and find that a gradual approach such as a guided body scan meditation or yoga *nidra* can be most helpful. I regularly practise this on days when I wake up more tired than when I went to bed, and it is incredibly restorative – the difference between functioning that day and not. Resting also makes my symptoms feel very acute at times, as I try to be present with it all.

I definitely had to learn to meditate as a practice. That still only works sometimes. It can be very hard to stop all the mental chatter, even when one's body is totally exhausted. The yoga practices, even if not always easy to totally focus, have remarkably changed me so I can quieten into a slower, calmer state of being.

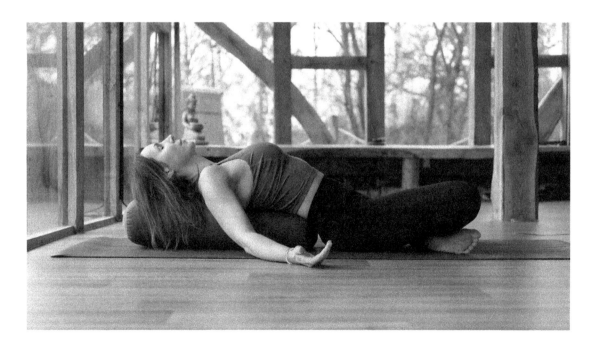

What do we learn from these comments? That rest doesn't come easily, but that it is very important to cultivate and prioritize. We also see that being still when there are difficult symptoms or a history of trauma can be challenging. And that a gentle yoga practice is an effective way of leading us into a deeper state of rest.

It's helpful to reframe rest as an *act of kindness towards ourselves*, and in our journey of self-compassion (see Chapter 10), this must be the foundation for healing. In a yoga teaching context, co-regulation from an authentic heart connection to the therapist alongside the ability to feel held in a safe loving space profoundly encourages the deep relaxation and sense of safety that is needed for healing.

DISCOVERING MEANING AND PURPOSE THROUGH REST

A definition of health, according to yoga, is to live a life where we can express our *dharma*, or our true purpose. What this means is that we are living in a way that is in sympathy with our authentic self. For example, if we are creative, we are able to express this. If we love nature, we make time to enjoy being outside, or even find work accordingly. If, however, we are living a life that is not in alignment with who we really are, yoga suggests that this will affect our wellbeing and may contribute to making us ill and stressed. So, if you are a banker in the City but would rather be a musician or gardener, you are not yet expressing your purpose, or *dharma*. You may resist this concept, by saying 'I don't know who I really am, or what my purpose in life is, and furthermore, I don't have the luxury of health, time or money to think about this kind of thing!'

Yoga is an active process that encourages us to discover our *dharma* through self-inquiry and contemplation, and for this we need proper relaxation, space and rest. This helps us to see the patterns and habits that cause our suffering with honesty and courage. As we saw earlier in the book, some of our conditioning, such as pushing through discomfort, or needing to constantly achieve, may cause us challenges. However, if we can see the root of these patterns, which very often comes from childhood, we can harness our new insight to help us to break our more destructive habitual way of being, so that we are no longer separated and distracted from peace. Contemplation shows us that it's possible to cultivate a happier life by incorporating new and different patterns such as proper rest, relaxation, meditation and pacing into our lives – both during and after illness. These are lifetime habits that will serve for a lifetime of health. The gold that we are looking for as we learn to slow down and become more still is our true self, or that which is not affected or identified by illness or any external experience. This is how our recovery starts and, with a bit of luck, this is how our *dharma*, or purpose, becomes apparent.

When we are no longer on autopilot we see that we have some choice in the way we make decisions. We discover that we are someone else beyond our illness, and that we don't need to identify as a sick, ill person anymore. Life may be different, but in many ways it is better than before, because illness has taken us out of the cultural systems that keep us imprisoned. We cannot unsee what we have now become aware of. As we become more conscious, we may realize how, in Western society, we are judged by what we do, what we produce and by what we own. We may start to question if this is right and if this is how we want to live. We may realize that there is actually something more valuable in life, as we explore what really matters. As we enjoy more quiet times of reflection, we become more empowered as we practise the art of resting in silence, and this brings us more hope, resilience and optimism, as we see purpose just in our simple daily existence. Living more authentically and connecting to others from the heart, being more present and more accepting of how things are in this moment, gives us a sense of meaning and contentment that we didn't have before. A regular yoga practice that incorporates deep rest can help to lead us to this.

THE CHALLENGES OF RESTING ON OUR JOURNEY TO RECOVERY

On this road to recovery we may, at times, feel overwhelmed. This will include frustration at the unfairness of being unwell, anger at not being able to do the things we once did, and fear of relapse, reinfection or of never getting better. We may feel isolated, ashamed, lonely and afraid but too ill to go out and meet people and to get the social connection that we need. At times, our symptoms may be so unpleasant that we fear the actual body itself, feeling that it has let us down. We may then spiral into more fear as we add in negative thoughts about our symptoms, imagining the relapse ahead, which, in turn, makes the symptoms worse. The fatigue and pain may, at times, seem terrifying and never-ending. We yearn to be back to 'normal'. Reading through this book, however, we hope it becomes clear that a new and better 'normal' is possible.

ACCEPTANCE

It's important on this journey that we learn to manage expectations. Healing and the pathway to recovery are not linear. Allowing ourselves rest and relaxation doesn't mean an immediate end to our symptoms, but it does mean cultivating a different relationship to them, and is a big step in the right direction. A regular yoga practice that includes an acceptance of our current state, however challenging, helps us to see that we no longer need to be in battle with our bodies, at war with our wounds. Allowing ourselves to feel awareness and curiosity for our symptoms encourages self-compassion, meaning that we can honour the entirety of our experience.

THE IMPORTANCE OF GRATITUDE – SEEING LIFE'S GLIMMERS

Encouraging gratitude as we heal, and celebrating each change as it happens, no matter how small, is an important step on the journey to recovery. The expression 'glimmers' was coined by Deb Dana, a licensed clinical social worker who special-izes in complex trauma. In her 2018 book *The Polyvagal Theory in Therapy*, she explains that our nervous system is greatly helped when we look for glimmers or small, positive things throughout the day. Glimmers can be thought of as moments of regulation for the nervous system, as opposed to triggers, which are moments of dysregulation. Examples of glimmers could be enjoying the sun shining, pausing for a cup of coffee or tea, stroking a pet, or just enjoying a beautiful view. These are very simple things that bring a slice of joy that we can focus on, notice and be grateful for. These glimmers actually help to rewire the brain (Hanson 2013; Hanson and Mendius 2009) into a default state of contentment, unlike the more dramatic activities that trigger our dopamine levels – such as social media or shopping – which are highly addictive. The practice of looking for glimmers is *not* about seeking happiness or striving only for a positive mindset, but rather about seeing joy in the small things around us, and being grateful for them. For there *is* much joy to be found, even in minor ways, every day. We realize this is not always easy. Sometimes when we are unwell, and things feel tough, it becomes much harder to see the glimmers that encourage us to have gratitude. When we connect to these small things, however, we create a sense of contentment, not just in our heads, but one that infuses as a full body experience, and this helps us feel more present, as we move more into sensation, coming out of the stuckness of our busy, chattering minds. In other words, looking for glimmers every day and practising gratitude as a result is really good for our wellbeing and mental health.

Keeping a gratitude jar

We suggested the idea of looking for glimmers on our restful yoga Facebook group, and one client with Long Covid shared her gratitude jar experience. Every time she has a glimmer, she writes it down and puts it into a special jar. Whenever she needs, she pulls out and reads the slips of paper from the jar to lift her spirits. She explained that she finds this very helpful. This was taken up by many in the community who have also found great solace in looking for glimmers and having a gratitude jar. We share the idea here as a helpful tip for others.

LET'S PRACTISE: Seeing the glimmers

1. The invitation, as always, is to sit, lie down or get comfortable in any way that feels right.

2. Gently allow the breath to settle, encouraging a low, slow and subtle breathing rhythm by placing a hand on the belly and feeling the soft rise and fall. With each out-breath, have a sense of letting go.

3. Notice the way your body responds to this softer way of breathing.

4. Observe how your body feels, from the top of your head to the soles of your feet.

5. Just reflect for a moment on this sentence without judgement, knowing you don't have to do anything with it: 'I accept this moment as it is now.'

6. Even if that's not true, there may have been a time when it was. Sometimes we forget this, and we move on to wishing for the next thing, which can distract us from what we are experiencing now. If we can, we cultivate an awareness of our current experience, accepting and allowing it, just as it is even when we feel tired, fatigued and unwell. If the acceptance of this moment is difficult for you to access, however, we invite you to remember something pleasant.

7. Think about a situation that makes you feel happy. This might be something small such as holding a cup of hot tea, sliding into the warm bath, walking in nature, greeting your dog or cat first thing in the morning, seeing friends, walking on the beach, the feeling of the sea or the sand between your toes or looking out of a window towards a blue sky.

8. Connect with one thing that resonates for you and notice how that makes you feel.

9. Notice how your body feels now. Notice any spaces of softness.

10. Try not to analyse anything; instead, focus on your body and the sensations and feelings with curiosity.

11. Maybe there's a quality attached to what you are feeling? Maybe there's even a colour or a scent. Perhaps there's a shape to this feeling. Allow yourself to observe this, without judgement.

12. Even if there is a sense of sadness – let that feeling be there. Or perhaps you sense resistance – let that also be there. All feelings are welcome.

13. Allow and accept all feelings, if possible, in the same way as you accept the clouds in the sky. Just notice them, allowing them, letting them be.

14. Come back to that feeling of awareness of the small joy or happiness you focused on earlier.

15. See if you can fully step into that experience and make it more vivid.

16. Again, notice the sensation, the warmth, the temperature around you, the colour and the light.

17. Perhaps you notice how subtly these feelings affect your heart. If you can, find gratitude for having this memory, encouraging the ability to change how you feel. This is how we can move from one sensation to another, by seeing and remembering the glimmers.

18. You can stay with this feeling for as long as you wish. Give space to it. There's no need

to try to hold on to it or change it, just allow it. Know that this can be something you can come back to at any time you need.

19. Placing one hand on your heart, allow this to be a reminder throughout the day that you can come back to this feeling whenever you want. Feel a sense of peace and connect to that sensation. When you are ready, come back into your body. Feel your feet in contact with the ground.

YOGA *NIDRA* FOR REST

Yoga *nidra* is a deep relaxation technique that gives the body a huge rest. It is said to be equivalent to up to four hours' sleep, so is extremely restorative, especially if there are problems with insomnia. Yoga *nidra*, also known as yogic sleep, is also an ancient practice used as a guide towards self-realization. This means to know who we truly are. Behind the chatter of the mind and the distractions of the emotions we find something that is ever-present and unchanging. This is our true nature, also known as *sat-chit-ananda* (existence, consciousness, bliss). As we rest with the coming and going of our thoughts and emotions, and as they start to settle, we may realize that there is something ever-present and deeply still behind all the noise. This may lead us to ask 'Who Am I?' as we see that we can't be our thoughts and feelings because they are always changing. This is not a question to answer here, but is for you to discover for yourself. This describes the more spiritual aspect of yoga. However, self-realization may not be for everyone, and many would rather benefit from yoga as a healing modality. Yoga *nidra* also gives a way to deeply relax as the practice draws attention inwards through a guided rotation of awareness of parts of the body.

To practise yoga *nidra*, first make yourself fully comfortable, lying down supported by cushions, covers, eye masks and anything you need to feel as comfortable as you can in your space. Your body temperature may drop as you rest, so please be warm enough, using blankets and socks if necessary. Make sure that you won't be disturbed, and keep as still as you are able to during the practice.

LET'S PRACTISE: Yoga *nidra*

1. Take a few moments to settle down, allowing the body to rest in a way that is easeful.

2. Make any adjustments as necessary, moving in ways that help the body to find a supported and restful position. Bring awareness to the breath (as long as this feels comfortable for you; if not, use your Safe Resource, or focus on the parts of the body in contact with the ground). Bring your awareness to the belly, inviting the breath to move up and down in a slow, rhythmic way. With each inhale and exhale, as you invite soft, quiet (which is slow and low) breathing, become aware of the breath as a form of loving kindness to yourself. Take a few moments as you settle into this rhythm of soft navel breathing. As you continue to settle into breathing, allow every inhale to invite a sense of energy and vitality, and each exhale a sense of release. At any time, if following the breath becomes uncomfortable, come back to your Safe Resource.

3. You are going to repeat a few words of self-compassion now, before you begin an exploration around the body. You can repeat the following as a silent *mantra*, a whisper, or perhaps out loud: 'My mind is peaceful, my body is peaceful.' Repeat this silently to yourself a few times. If you have another phrase that you use as your intention, please feel free to use that. Come back now to the awareness of soft belly breathing.

4. We now begin a rotation of awareness around the body. Focus on each part of the body as you hear it, but then move on to the next part. If you hear outside disturbances, let that be part of your experience and come back to the voice that is guiding you with this practice. Bring your awareness to the right hand. Right-hand thumb, right index finger, middle finger, ring finger and little finger of the right hand. Awareness now of the palm, back of the right hand. Sensing now the whole of the right hand. Forearm, elbow, right shoulder, whole of the right arm. Right side of the neck, chest, rib cage, right side of the belly, hip, right buttock, thigh, knee, shin, calf, top of the foot. Explore the skin on the top of the foot. Big toe, second toe, third toe, fourth toe, little toe. All the toes together. Sole of the right foot. Top of the foot. Whole of the foot, whole of the right leg, become aware of the whole right leg and foot. Right side of the torso, become aware of the right torso, right arm, whole of the right arm, right side of the body – the whole of the right side of the body. Right shoulder, right upper back, right lower back, whole of the back, whole of the right side of the body. Become aware of the right side of the body.

5. Now to the left. Bring your awareness to the left-hand thumb, left index finger, middle finger, ring finger and little finger of the left hand. Awareness now of the palm, back of the left hand. Sensing now the whole of the left hand. Forearm, elbow, left shoulder, whole of the left arm. Left side of the neck, chest, rib cage, left side of the belly, hip, left buttock, thigh, knee, shin, calf, top of the foot. Explore the skin on the top of the foot. Big toe, second toe, third toe, fourth toe, little toe. All the toes together. Sole of the left foot. Top of the left foot. Whole of the foot, whole of the left leg, become aware of the whole left leg and foot. Left side of the torso, become aware of the left torso, left arm, whole of the left arm, left side of the body – the whole of the left side of the body. Left shoulder, left upper back, left lower back, whole of the left back, whole of the left side of the body.

6. Become aware of the jaw. Be aware of the chin. Lower lip, upper lip, inside the mouth. Be aware of any taste of sensation in the mouth. Now the space below the nostrils.

Left nostril, right nostril. Bridge of the nose. Right cheek, left cheek, right eye, left eye, right eyelid, left eyelid, whole of the right eye area, whole of the left eye area. Right ear, left ear. Right temple, left temple. Whole of the face, whole of the face. Back of the head, the neck. Become aware of the whole of the head and neck. Now bring your awareness to your whole body, your whole body. Become aware of your whole body and the space around you. The whole of the body, the whole body. Now just be aware that you are supported by whatever you are lying on. Feel your soft support holding you.

7. Bring your awareness to the centre of the chest. Your heart space – whatever that may mean for you. Resting your awareness at your heart space, just focus on the heart space. Bring a sense of compassion to this soft heart space, a sense of compassion and even love.

8. You can choose to listen to these words, repeating them silently, or whispering them to yourself: 'I have ease in my body, I have openness in my heart, I am enough just as I am.'

9. Repeat these words a few times to yourself, observing their meaning for you, noticing the response in your body without judgement. Maintain awareness of the heart space and take some time in silence, giving space for resting, softening and observing the gentle belly breathing. [3 minutes of quiet]

10. Become aware of this restful breath, the easeful, effortless way in which the body breathes at rest. Visualize yourself, resting here, in this space. Sense this body and become aware of how deeply rested and rejuvenated this body is now.

11. Repeat silently three times: 'I have compassion and acceptance for how I am right now and this allows me to be present in this body. I am enough as I am.'

12. Slowly, start to bring awareness to the edges of your body. Become aware of the space around you and the parts of your body in contact with your support. Be aware of your skin as a safe container for your body. Bring your awareness to the sounds you can hear; notice the furthest sound you can hear outside the room. Become aware of the nearest sound you can hear. Notice the sounds the body makes at rest. Be aware of any sensation in the body such as a taste in the mouth or a scent in the air. Feel the touch of your clothing against your skin and the temperature of the air around you. Become aware of how it feels to be fully supported in this space. Gently start to roll the head from side to side. Wriggle your fingers and your toes. Make small movements with your body and start to stretch. When you are ready, roll to one side and stay there for a moment or two. Slowly come to sitting, rub your hands together and softly hold the palms over the eyes. When you are ready, open your eyes and remove your hands. Look around your space to bring you back to the here and now.

DEVELOPING A REFUGE OF QUIET

Like deep relaxation, regular periods of meditation can gently reprogramme our more stressful conditioned patterns of constant doing, busyness and rushing. Meditation helps to regulate the CNS, taking us out of chronic stress patterns, so that we find it easier to both rest and to pace ourselves. If we can have a daily practice of mindful attention in the present moment using relaxation, meditation, breathing or a yoga *nidra* practice, our default setting eventually comes back to its natural place of peace. In this way, we find inner strength and resilience, even when life is challenging, because we see that our true nature is always peaceful, whatever is happening externally, even in times of chaos, change or difficulty.

Many people think that meditation is about forcing the mind to be still as we sit in an uncomfortable position without moving for long periods of time. We see things rather differently. We find the most effective way to meditate is to relax as much as possible, sitting or lying, while allowing everything to be as it is. This means being still with whatever is happening in the present moment, even if the mind is racing, or if there are difficult symptoms, without judging sensations or emotions as they arise. By trusting the inner silence rather than trying to control or solve things, our intuition and way of the heart are revealed. This is how we can cultivate more peace as we let go of trying to micro-manage and control everything.

Practising yoga before we meditate helps to set the stage for this inner quietness. Thus, slow breathing, *mantra*, relaxation and mindfulness during a yoga practice are very important staging points. In terms of yoga philosophy, a practice helps us to become more *sattvic*, meaning that a lightness of being, together with mental clarity, arises towards the end of a yoga session, making it easier to find stillness in our meditation.

Why should I bother to meditate?

There is ample research to show that those who meditate regularly have more energy, compassion and a calmer state of mind (Valk *et al.* 2017). As we sit quietly and observe the mind, we learn how to accept that which cannot be changed and are able to take this attitude off the mat and apply it to our everyday lives. Thoughts, emotions and opinions may arise, even pain and fatigue, but if we are meditating regularly, we don't get so involved – we know everything always passes. On this inner journey of self-discovery, we find that we can reflect and respond rather than react when we are triggered. As our practice develops, we discover how to apply discernment and detachment to difficult situations in life. This is because we view our experience with more acceptance, calmness and spaciousness, rather than having a knee-jerk reaction to circumstances that challenge us.

LET'S PRACTISE: Gratitude meditation

The following practice helps to encourage a sense of gratitude and appreciation for what we have in life, rather than for what we don't have. As the mind becomes more single pointed and less scattered, it is reframed to have a more constructive outlook, which is so important for recovery. We begin by choosing a point of focus for our meditation such as the breath, or a concept such as loving kindness or compassion.

1. Lie down (or sit, if that's more comfortable for your breathing) in any way that helps you to relax. Use cushions, blankets or an eye mask, if you need to. Take a moment or two to arrive in your body. Now have a sense of being cosy as you snuggle and nest down into your support.

2. Visualize a hole next to you and imagine that you are letting your thoughts go out of your head, into the hole and down into the earth, to be held safely until you need them again. Let them go on every exhalation. Remind yourself that you don't need to think for now – you can come back to your thoughts later. If thoughts still arise, that's fine, just notice them and let them go without becoming involved.

3. Now imagine a cord (it can be like an umbilical cord) going down from your belly deep down into the earth, bringing you a sense of strength and grounding. Take your time to visualize this. As you inhale, breathe up nourishment and vitality from the earth through the cord. As you exhale, visualize breathing down the cord, letting the earth take away anything you no longer want.

4. Next imagine a soft cloak, made of any fabric you would like to choose. Picture the colour of the cloak, and the weight of the material. Imagine you are settling the cloak around you for protection, bringing safety and security to your whole being.

5. Drop your awareness into your body. Take a moment or two. Bring your awareness to your heart centre. Think of someone you are grateful for. This may be a pet or a person, such as a teacher, a guide, a friend or a relative. Bring this sense of gratitude to your heart. How does this feel? Rest for a moment, developing a sense of love and gratitude. Opening your heart to appreciation can be challenging, so you if can't feel this yet, don't worry – just focus on the feeling of the physical area around the heart.

6. Stay with this sensation for a few minutes. If the mind wanders, that's okay – just bring it back gently to the sense of gratitude and appreciation. You may like to think of some other things instead that you are grateful for today.

7. Observe stillness around you like a bubble of silence. Sensations come and go, but the silence is always there. If it feels okay, take your awareness and rest in the inner silence for some time. If this feels challenging to access, take your awareness to the natural pause after the exhale. Stay here for 5–10 minutes, focusing on the silence, or on the breath, if you find that easier.

8. Coming back to the body, visualize that you are inhaling and exhaling through your heart centre for 10 slow breaths. If you are not comfortable following the breath, leave this part out.

9. When you are ready, open your eyes, stretch and move a little. Take your hands to your eyes, cup your palms softly over them and slowly open and close your eyes a few times. Relax your hands back, so that you are ready to get on with your day. Or if you prefer, you can continue to rest.

LET'S PRACTISE: Finding peace in nature

This practice invites us to visualize a sense of grounding from nature.

1. Find a comfortable lying position. Closing the eyes if appropriate, begin to tune in to the movements of your body or your breath.

2. Visualize that you are walking down a mossy path in a beautiful wood. Your feet are bare and the ground feels warm, soft and comforting under your feet. Explore your wood – the spring buds unfurling on the trees, the sounds of birds, the smell of the wood mould. Feel the touch of fresh air on your skin. In the distance you can see a blue shimmer of bluebells.

3. Imagine that on your back you are carrying a rucksack. Just imagine how this feels. How heavy is it?

4. You come to a clearing in the woods. The sun is shining and there is a fast-flowing river with a mossy seat nearby. You stop at the river and unpack your rucksack, throwing the contents into the river. These are all the things you no longer want in your life. Enjoy the sense of unburdening yourself. You watch as the river takes everything away, taking them out of sight.

5. Imagine that you are now lying down on the mossy earth, feeling refreshed and lighter than before. Smell the scent of the river and listen to the sound of the water. Listen to the birdsong. Take a moment or two to explore the sense of the ground beneath you, the feeling of the earth supporting you. Say three times to yourself: 'In this moment, I let go, I am at peace.'

6. Now reflect: 'What brings me peace? How can I bring more peace into my life?'

7. Take your hands to your heart and on the out-breath slowly chant 'Om shanti' or 'Peace' for up to four breaths, either chanting out loud or silently to yourself.

8. Observe the stillness from the chant and the practice. Take a few minutes in stillness, just focusing on the breath or on the sensation of your feet whenever the mind wanders. When you are ready, slowly roll to one side and come up to sitting.

KEY POINTS

✓ Deep rest is very important to healing. This is especially true during the time of an active infection.

✓ Both the CDC (Centers for Disease Control and Prevention) in the USA and the National Health Service (NHS) in the UK recommend rest during Covid-19 to decrease the risk of Long Covid. They also suggest resting regularly to manage Long Covid.

✓ Rest can be defined as something that is restorative, intentional and relaxing.

✓ Stopping regularly to take deep rest allows the nervous system to restore.

✓ Many with Long Covid find resting difficult. This may be because of an addiction to stress hormones that keep us in the 'doing' mode, fear of boredom and patterns of perfectionism, pushing through and trying to please others.

✓ We can reframe rest as an act of kindness to self.

✓ Yoga, which includes deep rest, can help us to discover our *dharma*, or true purpose and truth in life.

✓ Self-inquiry can help us to see the root of our more destructive patterns such as why we feel the need to compete, push and achieve.

✓ Developing new habits (*samsakras* in Sanskrit), such as regular rest, relaxation, meditation and pacing, will serve us for a lifetime of health.

✓ In Western society we are judged by what we produce, what we do and what we own. However, although we think this is where happiness lies, it may lead to ill health and dissatisfaction.

✓ Long Covid can give us the opportunity to find more joy and meaning in just simple daily existence.

✓ An acceptance of how we are in every moment, even if there are difficult symptoms, is very helpful.

✓ Encouraging gratitude as we heal is important. For this, we can look for 'glimmers' in our life. These are the small, positive things that we find throughout our day, such as a moment in nature or a kind conversation.

✓ Looking for glimmers helps to regulate the nervous system.

✓ A yoga *nidra* practised regularly gives the body a huge rest.

✓ Regular periods of meditation can help to reprogramme our conditioned response of busyness and 'doing' all the time.

✓ We can meditate by relaxing and allowing everything to be as it is. In this way we practise non-resistance, even during times of difficulty.

✓ Slow breathing, chanting, relaxation and mindfulness are staging points to meditation.

Chapter 9

THE WISDOM OF THE BODY

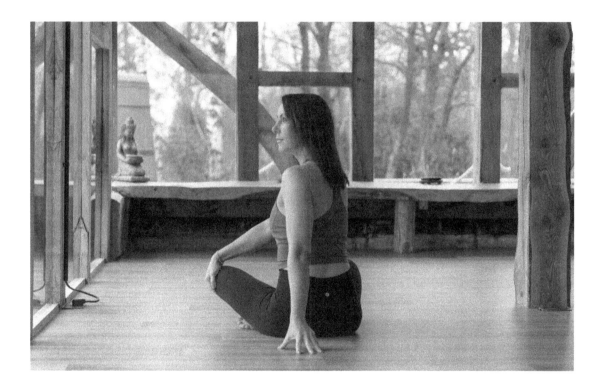

When we are managing the many expressions of Long Covid and fatigue, we may feel that we are battling our whole system, with each day offering a new symptom to navigate. The art of listening to how our body is feeling, however, is one way in which we can learn to understand the infinite healing wisdom that our bodies hold. The phrase 'listen to your body' is often used in a therapeutic yoga practice to encourage us to slow down or to stop when we are injured, exhausted or just not feeling good. Paying kind attention to how the body actually is means that we are then less likely to force, push through or ignore those sensations that tell us to rest. Recovering from illness requires us to cultivate a healthier relationship with our physical self, where we can track the subtle signals and cues our body gives *before* we feel like we have gone over the edge into relapse. As we learn to listen in, we also learn how to change the state of our nervous system by understanding how to pace and how to be kinder to ourselves.

Psychiatrist and trauma researcher Dr Bessel van der Kolk confirms this as he advises that, according to neuroscience, the only way we can change how we feel is in becoming aware of our inner experience, and learning to befriend what is going on inside (van der Kolk 2015).

HOW YOGA HELPS US TO CONNECT WITH OUR INNER WISDOM

Yoga therapy that encompasses breath, *mantra*, mindful movement and meditation can bring us closer to our source of wisdom, and this begins with the felt sense of the body. Finding this, however, means we must actually *inhabit* our bodies. We have already discovered in earlier chapters that, because of stress, trauma and a hectic pace of life, it is very common to dissociate from the body and to block internal cues from our awareness. We are not talking here about obsessive monitoring of all our symptoms. Rather, we need to feel our pleasure and pain, and also our more difficult emotions. We need to know whether we feel safe or unsafe, when it's okay to be vulnerable, and when we need to set boundaries. We can only do this by learning to listen in and trust our inner knowing. Unlike our minds, our bodies live in the present moment, and it is by noticing our body's language that we are able to become curious and consequently understand what our body is really saying to us. The more we listen, the more we come to learn that the body never lies and is advising us how to live more consciously. Ultimately, we want to welcome and be open to all our human experience and emotions as they arise, because when we repress and deny our more challenging sensations and feelings, we also close ourselves off from positive responses like happiness and joy.

INTEROCEPTION

Interoception means the ability to notice and understand internal sensations. This helps us to regulate the nervous system following chronic stress or illness by noticing, for example, when we are stressed, and when we need to rest. Previous life circumstances, however, may have altered this ability to listen in. For many, the pandemic caused us to detach from the present moment, as it seemed too frightening to be in the here-and-now. This consequently impaired our sense of trust in ourselves. The fear of being unwell, of family members being ill or of catching the virus, has increased health anxieties for many, challenging our interoceptive skills to uncomfortable levels. Unfortunately, a heightened state of anxiety and fear engenders a further sense of disconnection to our body or, conversely, encourages us to become overly vigilant of every sensation. Both scenarios activate the nervous system and increase dysregulation. Hyperawareness of bodily signals, for example, triggers anxiety, yet we may not read these signals accurately. Any small fluctuation in heart rate may result in excitatory messages to the brain, creating further unnecessary anxiety. This can lead to a loop of overwhelm, amplifying fear and panic. Equally, when we feel low, spaced-out and disconnected, we may experience exhaustion and emotional numbness, and so we detach yet further from our body's messages.

In our yoga practice, listening to the body is a skill we develop over time. This requires us to relearn interoceptive skills that we may have been conditioned to deny or repress. Take, for example, a child at school who may be told to sit when they need to move, wait to take a bathroom break and to not drink when thirsty, because of timetable constraints. The same can be said for going into work when we are unwell because of the pressures of financial commitments and the culture of our working environment that normalizes exhaustion. The health and fitness industry celebrates our ability to push through, with slogans such as 'Just Do It', which can, for some, mean exercising through injury, driving on through pain barriers and not taking adequate rest. We even see adverts for pain killers, encouraging us to go to work when we have 'flu. A trauma-informed yoga approach, however, supports the necessary process of relearning, befriending and listening to what the body is really saying in every moment, allowing us to gradually build trust in our body's messages again. This means we are more likely to act according to our wise internal cues rather than being influenced by external events.

INTEROCEPTION THROUGH SLOW MOVEMENT

In Western culture, the focus is often on sports and prescriptive movement. We move fast, getting to where we need to go as quickly as we can. However, yoga therapy cultivates mindful awareness of the current moment, and provides an excellent opportunity for us to hone essential interoceptive skills. So how do we do this? *By slowing down, going inside and noticing.*

Slowing movement down is an essential part of an embodied yoga practice. We want to become aware not just of the position in which we place our bodies, but also of the subtle sensations that arise inside. In other words, we want to become aware of the journey rather than the destination. We can ask ourselves questions such as: 'Am I forcing this movement, or can I back away from discomfort and find the "edge" of this feeling in which I can explore sensation?' And: 'How does it feel to move in this way?' When we allow ourselves to notice more than just the physical movement, we cultivate awareness of subtle, energetic sensations like tingling, warmth and feelings of spaciousness.

LET'S PRACTISE: Somatic awareness of the nervous system

This practice encompasses some of the ideas developed by Dr Peter Levine (2008), which explores the experience of being embodied in the present moment. All the practices do this to some extent, but here we use techniques that are designed to help us to increase an awareness of how it is to actually inhabit our bodies and that consequently help to discharge stress gently from the nervous system. From the yogic perspective, this is also about balancing *muladhara chakra* – our foundation – because it's a very grounding sequence.

1. Start by sitting comfortably. A dining or kitchen type chair is best – you want to be supported. Place your feet on the floor, or a cushion or block, and have your back against the back of a chair. Take a moment to welcome your current experience as much as you are able to. Notice any resistance as part of this process. Become aware of the feet, the connection of your body to the chair, and of your posture. Allow the spine to rise up softly, bringing space to the ribs and the place between the tailbone and the crown of the head. Rub your hands together and place them over your heart. Drop your awareness into your heart, welcoming yourself, and visualize light coming into the heart on every inhalation.

2. We are going to explore gravity and its relationship to your body. Start by becoming aware of the floor under your feet. Take some time here. Feel into the tops of the feet, then the soles. Explore the sensation of the surface under your feet. Notice any tingling in the feet and if they are warm or cool. Next, bring the weight of your body over your left buttock. Feel that you are pouring your weight down through the buttock, down through the left side. Take a moment or two to examine how that feels. Use the sense of curiosity to explore any sensation. Observe how your neck feels.

3. Now bring your weight back to the centre. Pause for a moment, then take your weight over to your right side. Again, pour your weight down through the buttock and lower body. Explore any sensation. Just play with how this feels. Come back to the centre. Next softly and very slowly sway from side to side, as if you are moving through syrup. Observe if the left or right side feels heavier, without making any judgement.

4. Come back to the centre. Slowly circle from your hips to make large circles with your torso. Explore this movement – make it slower, then faster, and your circles smaller, then larger. Then circle in the other direction. Be curious about what feels better.

5. Come back to the centre and pause, noticing how you are. Mind, body emotions, sensation and energy – how are they? Maybe these are all muddled but that's okay. Just observe without making any judgement.

6. Take the back of your right hand to your left cheek. Explore your cheek. How is the temperature? Is there any sensation there? Does the cheek feel soft or hard? How is the pressure? Now bring your awareness to the back of the hand. How does the hand feel? What is the texture? The temperature? Is there any tingling or sensation there? Take a moment or two to investigate these two surfaces – the cheek and the back of the hand, moving from one surface to the other.

7. When you are ready, drop the hand to the knee, pause and then repeat on the other side, exploring the feeling of the back of the left hand on the right cheek, just as you did before.

8. Pause for a moment, becoming aware of the felt sense of support of the floor and the chair. Feel that you are offering your feet to the ground like a prayer. Imagine roots going down from your feet into the floor and the earth below. As you inhale, draw up energy from the earth, nourishing you. As you exhale, let anything you no longer want to hold on to travel down the feet, down through the roots into the earth below. Have a sense of the earth supporting you.

9. Interlock your fingers and turn the palms inside out. Inhaling, lift your arms above your head. Take one in and out breath with the arms lifted.

10. On the next exhale, lower the arms, chanting 'Lam, lam, lam'. This is the seed *mantra* for the root *chakra muladhara*. If you don't want to chant you can just hum on the exhale as the arms float down, or remain silent.

11. Repeat slowly up to four times. If four is too many, do fewer repetitions. Now pause, resting the hands on the knees, and listen to what your body needs.

12. Inhaling, let your right arm float up, taking it next to the ear. Take a gentle side bend to the left. Come back to the centre. Inhale, then as you exhale, lower the arm down in time with the out-breath. Repeat this to the other side, this time bending to the right. Remember that no movement is right or wrong, so just explore how the body feels as you gently bend to both sides. You can bend further and hold for a few breaths, or remain more upright. Experiment with the movement. Notice the freedom created in the rib cage by the lifted arm. Investigate if one side feels different from the other.

13. Take your hands to *muladhara chakra* (the place around the base of the spine; if this isn't comfortable, you can visualize this area). With your eyes closed, take eight slow breaths, visualizing light coming into the base of the spine on every inhalation.

14. Now place your hands on your knees. Inhaling, lift the right arm out to the side, so it is parallel to the floor, following the fingers with your gaze. Exhaling, slowly float the right hand to the left shoulder. Take a few breaths as you massage your left shoulder. Inhale and take the right hand out to the right side again. Exhale and lower to the knee. Repeat this on the other side. Each time you massage your shoulder, have the sense that you are nourishing and taking care of yourself. When you have finished, rest with your hands on your knees.

15. Close your eyes, observing the softness of the inhalation and exhalation. Notice the effect of the practice on your whole being. Feel the support beneath you. When you are ready, stretch or move a little and carry on with your day.

SELF-INQUIRY

Most of us live in our heads for much of the time. Yet our minds are notorious for over-thinking, imagining, spinning stories, ruminating, micro-managing and worrying. Wrapped up with memories from the past, or planning and forecasting for an uncertain and sometimes frightening future, we consequently have a tendency not to be here, right now. We may find we are metaphorically imprisoned by the mind, reacting to life through our fears and desires. As we practise yoga, however, we become more curious about our inner experience. There is a very important concept in yoga called self-inquiry (*svadhyaya* in Sanskrit), which means being aware of and investigating the thoughts and patterns of the mind. Gradually, from this observation, we come to realize what is real and what is false. We may see that most of our patterns, including our judgements, our identities (such as what we do for a living, our class, race or even our illness) and our thinking in general, are actually part of an unconscious way of reacting to life. In time, as we become calmer, we may transcend the pairs of opposites that keep us trapped in habitual thought patterns of inner division and conflict. This includes our more entrenched opinions and polarization around certain ideas.

Self-inquiry in this context isn't quite the same as interoception, but listening to the body can be a portal or access point, as we learn to watch both the fluctuations of the mind and the sensations of the body with detached curiosity. As we go deeper (and we encourage you to seek support from a therapist as you do this), we may realize that our thoughts aren't actually real because they are always changing. For example, we may have a story that tells us we will never get better, or that we are useless or not good enough. With self-compassion and maybe some support, we can tenderly begin to dismantle this kind of fearful thinking. We need to practise this kind of self-inquiry with gentle discipline if we are to encourage the mind in a more helpful direction. Only when we are no longer prisoners of our more harmful patterns can we begin to heal. But first, we must explore our more unconscious shadow side. We can't dismantle the cage that keeps us stuck unless we understand and fully accept ourselves first. The dark as well as the light.

LISTENING TO THE BODY AND TAKING APPROPRIATE ACTION

When we listen in with greater awareness, we can better tend to our feelings and recognize behaviours that might otherwise hinder the recovery process. This means noticing our emotional state, or our posture, or inner narratives that might arise, as well as consciously attuning to the breath. For example, we can adjust our breath if we observe that we are hyperventilating, or we can pause and take time out if we see that we are going into overwhelm. If we realize that we are getting tired, we can stop. Learning when to stop is one of the most important steps in pacing, and knowing how to pace is a huge step in recovery. However, we can't pace effectively unless we first understand how to listen in with kind attention. As we move through the practices in the book, we are learning to take frequent pauses and rest between any movement. As we relax and become still, we can then apply our interoceptive skills by noticing the effects of the practice on the body, breath, mind, emotions and energy. This is witnessed with curiosity and not judgement. We then take this observation off the mat so that we can feel when we need to take a break during the day. In this way we avoid the boom or bust, tired but wired pattern, which is such a common scenario for those with Long Covid and chronic fatigue, by applying the wisdom of pacing. Pacing is such an important tool for recovery that we write more about it in Chapter 11. It starts, however, with the skill of interoception.

LET'S PRACTISE: Awareness of being

1. Sit or lie comfortably with as much support as you need.

2. Bring your awareness to the body. Become aware of the parts of the body in contact with the ground or support.

3. Sense the back of the body. Can you imagine drawing an imaginary line up your spine?

4. Become aware of your breath just as it is now. No judgement and no need to change anything.

5. What part of the body are you most aware of? Take some time to explore this, and remember that at any time you can come back to the sense of the support beneath you, or to your Safe Resource.

6. Do you notice any sensation in your back or legs? Warmth in your chest? Any sounds or movements in your belly?

7. If at any time you feel uncomfortable, come back to noticing the support you are resting on, the rhythm of your breathing, or your Safe Resource.

8. Become aware of the temperature of the skin – is it warm or cold?

9. Notice if you can feel the texture of your clothes against your skin, or the material under your hands.

10. Observe if certain areas of the body feel tense or restful and relaxed. Look for the differences between the upper body and lower body, then the left and right sides of the body. Don't judge or compare anything, just explore with curiosity.

11. Bring your awareness back to your breath. Is it shallow or deep? Do you feel the breath in your chest or low in your belly? Don't judge or label anything, just notice.

12. Bring awareness to the jaw, mouth, forehead and the muscles around the eyes. How does the expression on your face feel from the inside? Is there any taste inside the mouth?

13. Next, remember something pleasant, maybe a memory or a picture of something you like. It can be something small, like a sunny day, a hot cup of tea, perhaps a pet, or a starry night sky.

14. Notice now how your body and face may change as you think of this. Maybe your body softens with this idea.

15. Now remember something slightly unpleasant. This should be something mild that creates only a small level of discomfort. For example, a parcel not arriving on time, or an annoying fly in the house. Don't choose anything that is too challenging.[1]

16. Feel how your body reacts to this more unpleasant thought.

17. Go back and forth between these thoughts, noticing changes within the body and breath. Then pause. Just focus on the softness of your hands.

18. Slowly begin to feel your feet, or the parts of the body in contact with the ground or your support.

19. Begin to make small movements with your fingers and toes, and slowly open the eyes.

LISTENING TO THE LANGUAGE OF OUR NERVOUS SYSTEM

When we get curious about what our sensations are telling us, we can learn to regulate our nervous system better. For example, we can explore the following questions:

- Does the tightness in my chest arise in certain environments or around certain people?

- Does numbness or a zoning out show up when I start talking or thinking about certain things?

- Does my body language change when someone comes into the room, or when a particular emotion arises?

- What might these sensations be saying? Have I noticed this before, and if so, when?

---

1   We strongly encourage you to practise this exercise using only a mildly unpleasant thought or memory, and not to use anything which is traumatic. We recommend you always use a Safe Resource if, for any reason, a more difficult memory is recalled.

Asking ourselves these types of questions isn't about being self-absorbed, but is rather about being aware of the first subtle signs that are communicated by our bodies when we feel anxious, overwhelmed, nervous, reactive, tired and so on. When this happens, we can contemplate: 'What is it my body is telling me? And what action can I mindfully take?'

The consistent practice of noticing body sensations helps us to shift our nervous system to a more regulated place, by observing when we feel activated, so we can take gentle steps to adjust using breath, rest and movement, thereby promoting self-soothing and calmness. This has important implications for recovery because it impacts how we make decisions, how we engage with ourselves and other people and how we relate to the world around us. Every time we say 'yes' when our body is saying 'no', our nervous system finds a way to say 'no' for us, in order to slow us down, leaving us more susceptible to exhaustion, burnout or even illness.

LET'S PRACTISE: Body awareness for healing

Here, we examine how our bodily sensations might relate to different states of the nervous system using the model of Polyvagal Theory (from Chapter 2):

- Ventral vagal tone: in flow state, calmly energized (the *guna* of *sattva*)

- Sympathetic nervous system: also known as the fight, flight, freeze or stress response (the *guna* of *rajas*)

- Dorsal vagal tone: shutdown, freeze, dissociated (the *guna* of *tamas*).

  1. Sitting comfortably, close your eyes and feel your feet on the ground. If you can, think of breathing slow and low, through your nose. Take some time.

  2. Notice how you are feeling right now, with no need to change anything.

  3. Choose a word that describes that feeling. Perhaps it's 'happy', 'energized', 'tired', 'anxious', 'agitated', 'nothing in particular' or 'irritable'.

  4. Can you sense where this feeling or emotion related to the word is in your body? Encourage yourself to come out of your head and drop your awareness into your body so that you are now observing any sensation related to the emotion. Even if this doesn't make sense to you, allow the resistance to this concept to just be there, and notice what first arises as you sense into your body.

  5. Become aware of any sensations such as 'tightness', 'tension' and 'clenching'. These impressions would describe the state of being aroused by the sympathetic branch of the nervous system. Or you may feel 'happy and calm', in which case your nervous system is in a Ventral Vagal State. If you don't yet feel anything, that's also okay.

  6. As you observe with curiosity, also notice your posture, temperature and quality of

your breath, if you can. Place a hand on the part of the body relating to the sensation. If you can't find anything, that's okay. Witness all this without judgement. Everything is just as it is for now.

7. Sit for a moment longer and breathe into the space in your body that you may be aware of, inviting softness and warmth with each breath.

8. Observe the sensation, and if you can, bring a sense of kindness and expansion to the feeling – an acceptance of how it is just now. Try to feel what is happening as a physical sensation, rather than going into the mind and 'thinking' about it. Does it have a shape, a colour? Is it tingling or vibrating? Be curious about how the feeling is actually felt in the body.

9. Acknowledge the present moment by silently saying what is happening. For example: 'I am feeling anxious, and I can feel tightness in my chest' (if this is the case, this is an example of being in the sympathetic nervous system division).

10. Now, repeat to yourself: 'In this moment I offer softness and warmth to this area.'

11. Observe, without judgement or need to change anything, if the invitation of softness and warmth to this area changes the sensation. Allow yourself to just observe with kindness – continuing to breathe slow and low.

12. You may wish to invite awareness to other areas of the body by naming the feeling and observing it as a physical sensation. Take time to offer softness and warmth to these areas. Notice any changes, or resistance, knowing this is all part of the process of developing interoception.

13. Take your time to come back into the room or space that you are in. Feel the connection with your feet and the floor. When you are ready, softly open your eyes. Notice how you are. (If you feel calm, you may observe that your nervous system is now in ventral vagal tone, or more in the flow.)

LET'S PRACTISE: Sensing our inner experience

This next practice is about noticing our inner experience so that we can allow and even welcome all sensations and make the best choice in any given moment. It's about treating ourselves as our own best friend.

1. Gather blocks, bolsters, cushions – whatever is necessary to best support you. Remember, you don't need yoga equipment – there are many items in your house that can be used in place of these.

2. Sit or lie with your legs out straight in front of you. Next, bend the knees to bring the soles of the feet together creating a diamond shape with your legs.

3. Use blocks, or any other support you may need, under your knees.

4. This practice is not about how well you are able to hold the pose. Rather, it is about the awareness of sensation. Focus only on sensations.

5. Begin by becoming aware of the breath. Notice what it feels like to breathe. Observe where the breath goes. Can you follow the journey of the breath as it moves – such as at the nostrils, movement of shoulders, chest or belly? Can you feel the quality of the breath? Is it expansive or shallow? Does the breath feel smooth or ragged? Can you continue to keep your attention on the breath for the next 1–2 minutes?

6. Notice how the breath changes with time. Simply notice the changes.

7. Next, become aware of any area in the body where there may be tension. Can you take your focus there and become fully aware of the feeling? Is it deep or on the surface of the skin? Is it in one place or more than one? You might like to bring your awareness to your shoulders and your jaw. If you can't find a sensation anywhere, that's fine.

8. Direct your breath to this part of your body, feeling it soften and release more and more on every exhalation.

9. Next choose an area of the body where you feel the intensity of this position the most, such as around the pelvis, groin and hips. Again, just notice where this is. What is the sensation? Is it one place or more? Perhaps it has a shape or a quality? Is it warm or cool? Is it a constant sensation, or does it come and go?

10. Notice everything you can about this sensation. If the mind wanders, bring it gently back to the awareness of the sensation without judgement. If at any time this is too much, relax out of the posture by gently drawing the knees together.

11. Now, take your awareness to a sense of your internal state or inner feeling, if you are able to. Is there a particular emotion attached to the physical sensation? Is it uncomfortable, easeful or challenging? Is the urge to move or to stay still? Can you notice if there is a sense of this being good for you? A comfortable place to be? Or is moving out of the posture what is needed?

12. When you do decide to move, do so gently and with care, and remember not to force yourself to stay if it becomes tiring or challenging. Bring your knees back towards each other and gradually roll to one side. Remind yourself of the practice of moving with *ahimsa*, or non-violence to self.

13. Slowly and gently move your body, beginning at the fingers and toes. Take your time with each of the movements your body needs in order to release. Pause before you go back into your day.

KEY POINTS

- ✓ Recovery from illness requires us to cultivate a healthier relationship with the body as we learn to listen to our more subtle internal signals. This helps us to become more aware of our inner experience through a process called interoception.

- ✓ Life experiences and illness may create a sense of disconnection from the body. For many, learning to listen inward and connect with our physicality can be challenging.

- ✓ Hyperawareness of bodily signals can also lead to overwhelm and anxiety.

- ✓ Yoga therapy encourages slow, mindful movement to explore embodiment. This helps with the acknowledgement and realization of our present experience.

- ✓ Tools such as listening in with non-judgement and curiosity help us to slowly engage more with the body.

- ✓ Self-inquiry (*svadhyaya*) allows us to notice patterns and ways of thinking that may be keeping us trapped in habits that reduce our ability to heal and recover.

- ✓ Learning to listen to the language of our body means we can respond with compassion to ourselves. With practice this helps to shift the nervous system to a more regulated state.

Chapter 10

THE IMPORTANCE OF SELF-COMPASSION

CONVERSATION WITH A CLIENT WITH LONG COVID

Q: What was life like before Covid?

A: I was busy, always on the go. I had a full-time job, a family, and was training for my next half-marathon. I didn't really stop and I prided myself on managing everything. I would describe myself as a compulsive multi-tasker.

Q: So, what's the narrative in your head about people who do less than that?

A: If it's me, I see it as a failure, but if it's someone else, it's not. I think it's because I'm far harder on myself than on others.

WHY SELF-COMPASSION IS SO IMPORTANT

We have come to the conclusion that the biggest accelerator for recovery is the application of self-compassion. The biggest challenge to our health is *lack* of self-compassion. For most of us, however, the idea of any kind of self-empathy is extremely hard, yet we cannot make any meaningful progress without it. If we want to apply contemplation and self-inquiry as we journey towards healing, we can only do so successfully if we can cultivate a sense of compassion for ourselves.

WHAT DOES SELF-COMPASSION MEAN?

Self-compassion means a genuine consideration for ourselves that is at least equal to the regard we have for others. It means not pushing, not being driven and not needing to succeed, compete or achieve because of a lack of self-worth. It means deeply caring about ourselves, accepting ourselves as we are in each moment with tenderness, and treating ourselves like our own best friend. For many, these are difficult concepts because we (especially women) are brought up and conditioned to be of service, to always put others first and to think that it is egocentric and selfish, even narcissistic, to care for oneself. Yet the truth is, we can't look after and love others fully unless we love ourselves too. You may remember that the very first step in interoception is to become more *aware* of how we actually are in each moment and to notice what our thoughts are telling us. For this, we must apply self-compassion and non-judgement in our observation. If, however, we are thinking 'Oh goodness, I am so tired! Why are my joints still aching? My back doesn't feel right, I am so useless, I will never be well!' then that is going to add to our stress load and feelings of worthlessness. This is one of the reasons we discourage any form of competition or comparison in a yoga practice. It's just not compassionate.

THE INNER CRITIC

Many of us have an unkind voice in our heads that runs our life at a barely conscious level. The inner critic may tell us that we are useless, a failure, stupid, not good enough or too fat/thin/poor/old. Worse, it may tell us we will never get well. This voice is not an auditory hallucination, but actually a default mechanism of the nervous system designed to keep us (falsely) safe.

This inner critic often comes from internalized early life experiences that shape the way we think about ourselves, and could be described as thoughts and beliefs that oppose our best interests and diminish our self-esteem. Our inner critic encourages and strongly influences self-defeating and self-destructive behaviour, creating a pessimistic view of the world. The voice is often negative, simply because our brain has a negative bias and is metaphorically scanning the environment looking for threats, in order to take appropriate action for our survival. Because our system is wired to anticipate danger, there is a tendency to create fearful and critical thought patterns that can advise us when to fight or run. These thought patterns are a survival adaptation, but they can keep us locked in a stress response, as we focus on the worst-case scenario.

Many people worry that if they stop listening to their inner critic, they may lose touch with their intuition or conscience. However, unlike our true voice of the heart, the inner critic is not a trustworthy guide, and we need to understand the difference between the two. Rather than exacerbating the problem by criticizing our inner critic (which just makes us more stressed and sets up a vicious cycle), it's helpful if we can bring kindness to this internal monologue, recognizing that although it is trying to protect us, such pessimistic condemnation needs to be gently challenged with tenderness and empathy. It's good to talk to ourselves whenever we are aware of the critic as if we are our own best friend, or even a small child in need of some loving care and attention. Inner criticism may rear its head when we are practising self-inquiry, as we begin to see our unconscious patterns arise. We may blame ourselves, for example, for our more negative emotions, behaviours and addictions. What is much more helpful, however, is to see all of this with acceptance and compassion rather than with judgement.

LET'S PRACTISE: The cuddle breath

What's not to like about hugs? Hugs have a wealth of benefits. They boost oxytocin levels, leading to reduced feelings of anger, loneliness and isolation. Hugs raise serotonin, which improves our mood and helps to regulate our sleep cycle. Hugs release endorphins, the body's natural pain reliever. Hugs increase dopamine, helping to relieve depression. Hugs lower cortisol, which helps us calm the mind. They lower blood pressure, strengthen the immune system and alleviate tension in the body. The great thing is that we can have all these benefits by hugging ourselves. In the next practice, we show ourselves some kind attention and compassion with the cuddle breath. An added benefit is that by wrapping our arms around ourselves, we are also encouraging diaphragmatic breathing as we pacify the upper chest area with a very gentle, love-filled reminder to breathe slow and low.

1. Sit comfortably and bring awareness to your feet in contact with the ground or the support beneath you.

2. Notice the length of your spine, so the head, neck and spine are in line. Imagine space in the spine and a gentle sense of softness in the body.

3. Bring awareness to your breath.

4. Gently start to rock backwards and forwards, leaning forwards with your exhale, and curling backwards with the inhale. You may prefer to rock side to side, so experiment with both versions to see what feels best.

5. After a few breaths, bring your arms out about shoulder height, or wherever is comfortable, palms open as you inhale and lean forwards, and as you roll back and exhale, wrap your arms around your shoulders, taking the opposite hand to opposite shoulder to give yourself a hug.

6. Continue to move and rock in this way for a few more breaths, opening the arms on the inhale and hugging yourself on the exhale.

7. Slow the movement down and come to rest with your arms crossed over your chest, hands resting on shoulders.

8. Bring your focus back to the imagined line of your spine, and visualize space and softness in the body.

9. Breathe in a sense of peace for a few breaths on every inhale. Allow the felt sense of the hug to encourage a low, slow breath.

10. Experiment with what it feels like to slowly stroke down each arm with the opposite hand, as you continue to breathe slow and low.

11. When you are ready, feel your feet in contact with the ground and come back into your day.

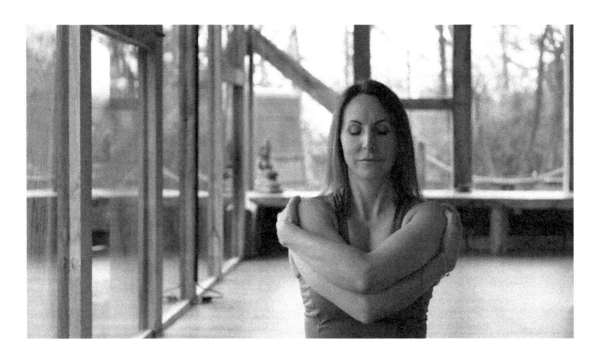

THE CHALLENGES OF SELF-COMPASSION

We appreciate that you may have very difficult life circumstances such as being a single parent, a carer for someone, or just trying to survive financially in order to pay the bills, mortgage or rent. Being kind enough to take micro-breaks and adequate rest in order to recover may seem almost impossible. The responsibility to others such as family, work colleagues and friends all too often means we ignore those interoceptive cues that tell us to stop. In our own recovery, we both have had to learn to pace, rest and stop when necessary. This is what it means to practise self-compassion: understanding the importance of boundaries, saying 'no', pacing not pushing, listening to the wise inner voice, challenging the voice of the inner critic, and applying self-care when necessary. This is the path to recovery.

LET'S PRACTISE: Becoming your own best friend with journaling

Often, we are better able to bring compassion to others while ignoring the need for kindness to ourselves. The following practice allows us to think of how we might treat others, and how we could consequently change the view of how we treat ourselves. After the practice, you may like to journal and reflect what came up for you.

1. Come to a comfortable position. Settle into the space and observe your body and breath. Take some time to reflect on the following questions:

   – Can you recall a time when a close friend was struggling with something, or perhaps felt bad about themselves? How did you respond? Think about the things you typically say or do in this situation.

   – Now, think about a time when you felt bad about yourself, or you were struggling with something. What would be your typical response? What can you imagine yourself saying to yourself in these circumstances?

2. Do you notice a difference between the two scenarios? Spend some time reflecting on, or writing down, how you could instead treat yourself in the same compassionate way that you'd treat your friend.

3. Be aware of the tone of voice that you use when you talk to yourself. Is this the same tone that you use with others? What language would a wise, nurturing friend, parent or mentor use? What is the most positive message you can give yourself that is in line with supporting yourself with love and care?

4. Take time to reflect upon the differences you noticed. You may wish to say out loud to yourself the same message you gave your friend. Notice how it feels to bring softness and kindness to your words for yourself.

5. Allow a moment or two to rest, knowing that, with practice, you can reflect kindness back to yourself.

THE IMPORTANCE OF KINDNESS AND LOVE WHEN APPLYING SELF-INQUIRY

The greatest gift we can give ourselves is to be open-hearted about our progress, especially on the more difficult days. When we are disconnected from ourselves and facing challenging times, it's helpful to bring our loving awareness to this, so we see we are in a state of distress and that suffering is not unique to us – it is part of the human condition and will eventually pass. We can maybe place a hand on our heart as an act of being with ourselves, or offer loving thoughts to ourselves, such as 'I am with you', 'I am safe', 'I love you', 'I have compassion for what I am going through right now' or 'This too shall pass'. With time and practice, cultivating self-support and kindness promotes more self-compassion. As we stop judging ourselves and our circumstances so harshly, we find that we also judge others less. This means we can radiate genuine understanding, compassion, peace and kindness outwards to our wider community, which is just what the world needs right now.

THE LADDER OF COMPASSION

Some people freeze or shut down when self-compassion is mentioned because it is so far from their experience. Therefore, we have to take baby steps. A yoga practice is an ideal place in which to cultivate more kindness to self as we slow down, listen inwards and make space to honour our inner rhythm. As we become still, we can explore what arises. Because we may find self-compassion difficult, we can work with a ladder of intention. We start by bringing *awareness* to and observing our inner voice. Are we in judgement? Are we resisting our current experience? Are we running an unkind, critical monologue? From this awareness, we can work towards *acceptance* by using the tools of curiosity and non-judgement to observe how we are in the present moment. Next, if we are able to, we apply a sense of *kindness* and also *spaciousness* to how we find ourselves. With time and with practice, we will eventually discover a sense of *self-compassion*. Finally, we may become aware of a genuine feeling of *love and deep caring from the heart for ourselves* and for our human experience, without judging anything as good or bad. It is just what it is. Even if there is pain, discomfort or exhaustion, we can bring kindness and love to this. So, our ladder is built of these rungs: *awareness, non-judgement, acceptance, spaciousness, kindness, self-compassion, love.*

THE FIRST STEP – ACCEPTANCE

Self-compassion starts with the art of acceptance. If you are not ready to apply self-compassion or love, see if you can work initially with awareness and maybe a sense of acceptance of how you are right now and for whatever you are facing in the moment. If we use self-compassion as a way to try to make our physical or emotional pain go away by either suppressing it, fighting against it or even faking it, things may likely feel more painful as we are just trying to bypass what is happening. What we resist will persist. We should try to remember that imperfection is part of the shared human experience, and that becoming mindfully more accepting of discomfort in each moment and embracing ourselves with care actually *is* an act of compassion. When we hold ourselves with acceptance and connection, we give ourselves the support and comfort necessary to bear the pain, while providing the optimal conditions for resilience, growth and transformation.

LET'S PRACTISE: Acceptance, kindness and love

In this next practice we focus on incorporating self-compassion into our experience. For this we are using the *bhavana* of love. *Bhavana* means focus, and it can be very uplifting to have a focus that we chant. Love is the quality of the heart, and we can explore and embody this more as the mind becomes quieter from the practice.

1. Come to a comfortable seated position. Take some time to arrive into your body, exploring how you are right now with curiosity. Welcome everything, resisting nothing about your current experience, if possible. How is your nervous system? Are you stressed in any way? For example: do you find it difficult to be present and engaged? Is the mind jumping about? Or are you relaxed and quiet? Welcome yourself however you are, allowing everything to be as it is. Bring in a sense of kindness to yourself in this present moment, if you can.

2. Explore your posture, taking some time to sense where the body is in the space you are in. Just observe without judgement.

3. Bring a sense of softness to your jaw and the area around your eyes. Imagine sunlight on your face.

4. Experience your breath. Where in your body do you feel it? Is it fast or slow? Notice how it is without changing the rhythm. Gradually encourage the breath to slow down, reminding yourself to breathe: slow and low and breathing through the nose, if you can. Be kind to yourself – if this is too much, that's fine. Bring compassion to however you are. If this is challenging, see if you can bring acceptance to your experience as it is right now, knowing that each day is different.

5. Inhale a sense of gentle sunlight to the belly. Exhale and pause for a natural count of one or two after the out-breath – if this is comfortable. There is no need to force anything.

6. Now feel soft sunlight flooding the body on the inhalation with the quality of healing energy. On the exhalation, allow everything to let go and become quiet. Try this for five breaths.

7. Stop to rest, breathe normally and observe stillness and peace.

8. If you would like, you are going to chant to the heart. Take your hands to your mouth to breathe into them, warming them, then rub the palms together and rest them over your heart. Inhale. Chant 'Om bhakti namaha' as you exhale, having a sense of chanting a soft loving lullaby to your heart. Try this three times. The meaning is: 'I am not separate from love.' If you prefer, you can chant 'Love, love, love' to the heart space, or you could hum on every exhale. *Mantra* protects and transforms the mind and helps to bring us to more positive states. Sound also increases circulation and helps to balance the *chakras*, bringing both vitality and peace. It is said that with regular practice, *mantra* also helps to pacify disease as the vibration clears away impurities.

9. Pause, reflecting on courage as the quality of the heart. Consider how you can bring more courage to your life. You might like to visualize the *mantra* physically being placed at the heart.

10. Gently sway from your seated position, moving the body from side to side. Explore how your body feels. Pause and become aware of the feeling of the inner body. Focus on energy as *prana* moving down the spine on the inhale, and on the exhale, the energy moving up.

11. On your next in-breath, starting with the palms together in prayer *mudra* at the heart, circle your arms out to the sides and then slowly bring the hands, palms together in prayer, above your head. Exhale and draw them back down to prayer at your heart. Repeat 3–5 times. You can chant 'Om bhakti namaha' if you would like on the exhalation, or 'Love, love, love', or you can just hum. Then sit quietly for a few breaths.

12. Inhaling, lift your right arm out to the side and up beside the ear. Pause, taking an inhale, and then exhale and another inhale; then on the next exhale, bend slightly to the left. Inhale, straighten the arm and centre the body, exhale and lower the arm. Repeat once more if your energy is all right, then do the same on the other side with the left arm as you bend gently to the right.

13. Rest with the hands on the knees and take a moment to observe how you are. How is your heart? Drop your awareness to your heart and observe.

14. Roll your shoulders slowly three times. Take your right hand to your left shoulder and massage your shoulder with a sense of compassion, thanking your shoulder for all that it carries. Repeat on the other side.

15. If appropriate, transition to come down onto all fours – knees hip width apart and hands under the shoulders with fingers spread, into a comfortable Cat position. Take your weight slightly over your knees, or bring the hands slightly forward if this is too strong for your wrists. Sense space between the crown of your head and your tailbone. Use any padding you might need under your knees such as a folded blanket. Remain seated, if you prefer. Inhale and lift the heart. Exhale and round the spine, dropping the head, taking the navel to the spine. Breathe and move like this 3–5 times.

16. If comfortable, sit back on your heels (you can place a block or cushion if your bottom doesn't come all the way down) and take your forehead to the floor, with your arms in front of you. A cushion can be used under your forehead to raise your head if it's more comfortable. Your knees are wide apart. Feel that you are surrendering your forehead to the earth. Relax down in this position. If this isn't comfortable, rest on your back or front. If you are seated, you can fold forward, allowing the head to hang down and then uncurl back up slowly when you are ready.

17. Come down to lying on your front. Bend your arms and rest your forehead on the back of your hands. (Arms are by your side and the head is to one side if more comfortable.) Take a moment or two to explore your breath from this position. Focus on moving the breath into your back – directing it into your back ribs, visualizing

the breath as light, as *prana*, filling you with healing energy every time you breathe in. Next, focus on gently expanding the lower ribs and belly onto the floor, feeling the soft pressure of the belly against the floor as you inhale. Have a felt sense of the ground supporting you.

18. As you exhale, hum the breath out, drawing the abdominal muscles in softly towards the spine. Take up to five breaths like this.

19. Bring the arms down beside the body, fingers pointing towards the feet, palms up. Inhale and lift first the right leg, lowering on the exhalation, and then the left. Don't lift too high – just a few centimetres off the floor, if that's not too much. Repeat three times to each side. Remember to be aware of your energy levels and do fewer repetitions if necessary. Be compassionate and listen to what your body needs.

20. Bring your hands up towards your shoulders and gently slide them forward, forearms to the ground, elbows under shoulders, like a sphinx, so that your chest is gently lifted off the floor. Your elbows are under your shoulders and palms are facing down. Keep your navel on the mat. The back of the neck is long with the chin slightly tucked in. Draw your shoulders towards your feet.

21. Inhale and look towards one shoulder, exhale, centre, and then inhale and look towards the other shoulder. Then come back to the centre. Keep the jaw released. Soften the eyes. Bring awareness to your breathing.

22. Come down on an exhale. Rest on your front for a few breaths.

23. The invitation is to now bend the knees and slowly sway them from side to side, so the soles of the feet are facing the ceiling. Explore how that feels. How does the back feel? The hips?

24. Slowly come up to kneeling in order to transition to lying on your back, if that's okay for your breathing. Otherwise come back to sitting. Rest for as long as you need.

LET'S PRACTISE: Cultivating courage

Courage comes from the heart, not the head, and is about listening to our intuition. It's about finding our inner truth, acting from that and paying less attention to external cues. In the last practice we focused on compassion and *bhakti* (love). In this next practice we are now turning this love back to ourselves. If you find this challenging, you might like to work with the idea of self-acceptance rather than love. But know that with time and practice, love and self-compassion will grow. We also use some gentle movement to help us to meditate and rest at the end of the practice.

1. Come to a comfortable sitting position. Allow yourself to arrive in the body. Take some time to settle. Take your hands to your heart and welcome yourself. Observe how you are. Allow everything to be as it is. Drop your awareness into the heart. If you have a question, ask your heart. Leave it in the silence.

2. If you are lying down, visualize the next movements. If you are sitting, softly lift your ribs and your heart, so that you are lifting and opening the front body, rather than collapsing over your ribs and diaphragm (our usual way of sitting because of the way we work these days). Just observe how you feel.

3. Feel a sense of the Earth beneath your feet.

4. Keep your hands on your heart with your awareness softly there. If you would like, you can chant 'Bhakti namaha' ('I am not separate from and I surrender to love') softly to your heart three times, or chant 'Love' if you prefer. You can also choose to remain silent and just breathe.

5. Courage comes from love. What we focus on we become, so now focus on a sense of courage in your heart. If you find this hard, think of someone or something you love who has strength, and imagine absorbing their strength and courage into your heart. As you do this, see if you can also focus on a sense of gratitude for what you have, rather than what you don't have. Focus on these qualities of love, gratitude and courage. Really imagine and feel these at your heart, if you are able to.

6. Feel that you are flooding your whole being with the idea of gratitude, love and courage. Know that you are not separate from love, and that this love is in you.

7. If you are sitting, come down to a comfortable lying position with the knees bent and have some support under your head.

8. Allow the shoulders to soften. Gently roll the head from side to side as slowly as you can. Allow the back to relax more and more with every exhalation, sinking into your support. Take one hand to the heart and one to the belly. Slowly and not too deeply, breathe into the hand on the belly, feeling the softness of the rise and fall with the breath. Think of the breath being slow and low. Think of the breath as your friend.

9. If you don't have back issues, when you are feeling fully relaxed, straighten out the legs, having them slightly apart. Rest and observe for a few moments. If comfortable, follow the gentle inhale and exhale through your nose.

10. Bring the feet together, then gently draw the knees over the belly. Take one hand to each knee (or you can hold under the knees if it's easier). Following the breath, inhale to let the knees float away from you as the arms straighten, and as you exhale, draw the knees in towards you. If you don't want to follow the breath, just do the movement. Repeat 3–5 times.

11. Now circle the knees apart and then back together. With a hand on each knee, inhale, pushing the knees away from you, and then let them widen. Exhale, draw them towards you, and then bring them together. Make about three circles like this, then reverse the movement, circling the other way. Focus on the massaging effect on your lower back, noticing where you are touching the mat with your back as the pressure changes.

12. Drop your feet to the mat with the knees bent, feet hip width apart. Rest for a few breaths, just observing how the mind, body and emotions are. Focus on the relaxing effect of the exhalation on the whole being – a long, smooth exhalation.

13. Bend your knees over your belly again. Inhaling, lift the right leg up, keeping the knee soft. Exhaling, bend the knee back to the belly. Inhaling, lift the left leg. Exhaling, bend it back. Repeat 3–5 times on each side, but really pay attention to your energy levels so that you are not pushing or competing with yourself. If you are tired, rest. Be compassionate, listening in to how your energy is. You can experiment by keeping the knee and the foot soft as you lift. If you want to move more dynamically, open the back of the knee and flex the foot as you raise the leg up. You don't have to lift too high – play with the movement and see what feels right.

14. Rest in a comfortable position. Observe how you feel, allowing the mind to settle and become still. Remember, we pause after any activity or movement in order to remind ourselves to pace and to give the system space to recalibrate. This is self-compassion in action.

15. Bend your knees, having your feet hip width apart and heels towards the buttocks. The palms are down beside the hips. Lengthen the back of your neck by gently bringing your chin towards the top of your chest.

16. Take an in-breath. Exhale and very gently take your navel to your spine to slightly tilt the pelvis. Relax on the inhale. Observe the movement of the pelvis as you breathe. Repeat 3–5 times.

17. Inhaling, press on your hands and feet to gently lift the hips to come up onto the shoulders, chin into chest so the back of the neck is long. Keep the knees stable. You don't have to come up too high, but as you lift up, have the feeling of lifting your heart. Take one breath here, then come down on a slow exhalation. If this is enough, rest, otherwise repeat twice more, always listening in and working kindly with your energy levels. Remember to pace, not push.

18. Draw your knees into your belly and rock out from side to side. Then finish by coming back into your relaxation posture.

19. Focus on the feeling in your heart centre. Ask yourself: 'What is it that brings me courage in my life? How can I bring this quality more into my life?' This is a reflective question for you to meditate on, so don't necessarily expect an answer. Just drop your question into silence.

20. Rest, focusing on the silence, for up to 5 minutes.

21. Stretch and move gently, and when you are ready, get up to continue with your day.

LET'S PRACTISE: Exploring self-compassion

In the last chapter we shared a practice that explored listening into the body when there was a manageable challenge present, using interoceptive skills. Here, we build on this idea by bringing in a sense of self-compassion.

1. Make yourself as comfortable as you can, sitting or lying. As always, you can access your Safe Resource at any time.

2. Think of a situation in life that is causing you just a little bit of stress. Please choose something that is not too overwhelming.

3. Using the tools we learned in the interoception practices, can you feel where any emotional discomfort is in your body?

4. Take some time to observe this as a felt, physical response in the body, rather than ruminating in the head. Explore any physical sensations. Bring your awareness back to your Safe Resource at any time if you feel the sensations are too much. If you can't feel anything, that is also fine.

5. Now say silently to yourself 'This is a moment of challenge'. You may wish to use a different phrase such as 'This is a moment of stress', or whatever best applies, just so you can be mindful of your current experience.

6. Now say to yourself 'I know that this difficulty will pass' or perhaps 'I am not alone'.

7. Resting your hands over your heart, feel the warmth of the hands and their touch on the heart centre.

8. Now say silently or aloud 'May I be kind to myself in this moment'. You may also wish to ask yourself: 'What is it that I need to hear to convey kindness to myself right now? What are my needs?' Finding a personal approach that speaks to you can take time, so remember to be patient.

9. Stay for a while repeating these phrases. Notice how it feels physically to bring kindness and warmth towards yourself. See if you can also bring a sense of spaciousness or light to the physical sensation, allowing it to be as it is.

10. Ask yourself: 'What is my inner self asking for?' This is a reflective question so doesn't require an answer now – you are just dropping this into the silence.

11. For many of us, self-compassion can be an uncomfortable process, and we may experience resistance. If you can, give yourself the space to explore how it feels to acknowledge this discomfort.

12. Rest for a few minutes. Observe if anything is changing. Come back into the body, and become aware of your feet and the base of your spine. Feel that you are inhabiting your body. When you are ready, move in any way that feels right, then carry on with your day.

KEY POINTS

✓ The biggest accelerator for recovery is self-compassion, but many of us find this hard.

✓ Self-compassion means a genuine consideration for ourselves that is equal in our regard for others.

✓ Self-compassion means not pushing or competing because of lack of self-worth.

✓ We should try to accept ourselves as we are and treat ourselves like our best friend.

✓ Many of us have an inner critic that runs us at a barely conscious level.

✓ This is a default of the nervous system to keep us (falsely) safe.

✓ It is helpful if we can be aware of our inner monologue and bring kindness and compassion to this inner voice.

✓ Self-compassion means understanding boundaries, knowing when to say no, pacing not pushing, and applying self-care when necessary.

✓ We can start employing self-compassion by bringing awareness to how we are in the current moment, using curiosity and non-judgement. Then, if we can, we develop acceptance of this, bringing spaciousness and kindness to anything that is difficult.

✓ With time and practice, we can develop love and deep caring for ourselves that comes from the heart.

Chapter 11

WHEN TO MOVE AND WHEN TO PACE

IS EXERCISE ALWAYS THE ANSWER?

When Nadyne was recovering from the acute phase of Covid-19, she was asked if she'd like to join a post-Covid running club. She had to laugh, as she was still experiencing severe breathing issues and chest pain. But then the laughter turned to concern. If she was being told that exercise would help her regain her energy, how many others were being told the same?

Many people with ME/CFS are still encouraged to engage in graded exercise therapy, despite the changes to UK guidelines made in November 2021. This is when the National Institute for Health and Care Excellence (NICE) (2021) finally removed the longstanding recommendations that patients with persistent fatigue should be prescribed graded activity as a treatment. The new guidelines make it clear that any programme based on fixed incremental increases in physical activity or exercise should not be offered for the treatment of ME/CFS (Vink and Vink-Niese 2022). The World Health Organization (WHO) rehabilitation guidelines for adults living with Long Covid are equally clear that 'exercise interventions should not be used in people experiencing post-exertional malaise exacerbation (PEM)' (WHO 2023).

UNDERSTANDING POST-EXERTIONAL MALAISE

Post-exertional malaise (PEM) refers to a significant worsening of symptoms and fatigue (or relapse) following physical, emotional or mental exertion. PEM and the triggers for it can be particularly challenging to monitor, especially on days where we sense we have more energy and so do more than we should. The type, severity and duration of symptoms following exertion may be unexpected or seem out of proportion to the initial provocation, which can be as mild as talking on the phone or being at the computer (Spotila 2010). As our energy improves, we may be encouraged to do too much, when the reality is that our body is still recovering. This can lead to a cycle of increased fatigue, muscle pain and cognitive impairment, which delays recovery further. We call this the 'push–crash' cycle. This is a very common scenario in Long Covid, and in this chapter, we explore how to break it.

Unfortunately, many Long Covid rehab programmes continue to be held in gym-based environments, supporting the idea that somehow exercise is the answer. Of course, physiotherapists and fitness professionals are doing their best to educate themselves about the potential negative effects of exercise on PEM and fatigue. Graded exercise therapy, however, is often poorly understood, and many well-intentioned healthcare professionals continue to advise those with Long Covid and CFS to build up their exercise tolerance in order to regain energy. Regrettably, there are numerous accounts of people advised to try 'Couch to 5km' – a progressive beginners running plan. *Research, however, is providing evidence that exercise is* not *the key to recovery, especially for fatigue-based conditions.*

For those used to a regime of regular physical activity, finding themselves unable to exercise can be intensely upsetting. The main method of regulating mental and physical wellbeing has been removed, further reducing the ability to cope with the stress of post-viral fatigue and the challenge of trying to get better. It's important to find acceptance of how we are in each moment, however, and that we remind ourselves this is *just for now*, that every day is different, and that there are other ways to help recovery that don't involve exercise.

We want to make it very clear that we are not suggesting you will never exercise again. We are, however, making the important distinction that when we are recuperating from an illness that depletes the body, dysregulates the nervous system and affects many of the major organ systems, exercise and forcing ourselves to continue to push on through is detrimental. This involves a shift in mindset and an understanding that we can see the benefits of exercise from a *different* approach to movement and breath, such as is offered by yoga.

WHY IS PACING SO IMPORTANT?

Fatigue is one of the most common symptoms of Long Covid. Unfortunately, the word 'fatigue' does not really convey the severity or chronicity of fatigue or its impact on daily life. Although fatigue is a common experience for everyone, persistent, unrelenting and profound exhaustion such as is experienced by those with ME/CFS, post-viral fatigue and Long Covid has no one particular physiological explanation. This means that there are as yet no objective markers for diagnostic testing (although we are hopeful that new research relating to the mitochondria will provide this soon), and so many people are left without any treatment plan and, in many cases, suffer from medical gaslighting.

Ron Davis, Professor of Biochemistry and Genetics at Stanford University, says: 'It's vital to know when you're at your energy envelope limit, and not to exceed it for any reason' (quoted in Prior 2021). We know personally how challenging this can be. Clearly, however, it is important to get very serious about energy limits and not gamble with the tempting idea of 'I'll do this now and push through, knowing I'll crash later, but I'm willing to take the consequences anyway'. Medical advice on pacing for CFS/ME is always to do half of what you think you can do, because the risk of feeling full of energy and then overdoing things and crashing is a very real possibility.

THE CHALLENGE OF SLOWING DOWN

We advise caution to anyone who is urged to increase their physical exercise too quickly. Rather, we suggest monitoring energy levels and *staying below the energy envelope* for the entire recovery period. In other words, *do less* than you think you can in order to conserve energy for healing. This doesn't mean never exercising or being active again, but it does mean that, for many, there is a need to reassess their relationship to 'exercise'. *This is very important.* First, if you are unaware of the push–crash cycle of PEM, you may inadvertently do too much of something beyond your current capacity. Second, energy levels in this population fluctuate hugely, and monitoring this is very difficult for the person with chronic fatigue. They may feel well on the day, and then do too much, leading to relapse, which may happen a few days after the activity that caused the crash. Finally, the person with Long Covid may override their body's messages and push themselves, regardless of their tiredness, believing that strong activity and a continuation of being in the 'doing' zone is the answer to recovery. We explored this in Chapters 1 and 2, where we saw how it is part of our culture to keep busy to the extent that we normalize exhaustion. Stress hormones can be addictive, keeping us in the 'doing' mode, whereas resting is challenging because it can initially make us achy and sore and seem very boring. Patterns are patterns, however, because they repeat, and although it may be hard to slow down, it's important to challenge our more unhelpful patterns as we move towards an understanding of how it feels just to 'be'.

So, gentle is the way forward, with the focus being on breathing, relaxation and just a little movement. *Remember, the application of functional breathing is actually, to our bodies and brains, more important than exercise in terms of oxygen uptake to the cell.* We need to make sure that we have micro-breaks throughout the day after any activity, to allow the body to recalibrate and restore. Breathing, resting and pacing are the best friends we can have in our healing journey.

Annabelle is a retired doctor. She worked successfully her whole life in busy hospitals around the world, so was distressed to find herself suffering intense fatigue following

Covid-19. Prior to her illness, she had been an active member of the community, singing in the local choir, busy caring for an elderly parent, and enjoying a full social life. After she had Covid-19, even walking her dog down the garden path was too much for her, and she resigned herself to days spent in a comfy chair. This, inevitably, made her depressed. She admitted that in the past she had dismissed chronic fatigue when it was mentioned by patients; she used to think they were lazy and just needed a good nap. She consequently felt that, in her case, it was very important to keep going but this, of course, hindered her recovery. Resting seemed such a waste of time, when there were things to do and people to see. On the days she felt a bit better she would rush back into normal life, walking the dog again and arranging to meet and care for friends and family. Eventually she realized this was keeping her stuck in a cycle of doing too much, as each relapse period got longer. With the help of a yoga therapist, she was able to recognize why her need to be busy distracted her from how she was really feeling, and how this had its root in a pattern going back to childhood. She was helped to reframe the desire to go back to her previous way of life too quickly, towards a recognition of what her body needed each day. She is now able to take rest and recovery periods by understanding her energy levels and how to pace, and she has slowly reintroduced activities that bring her joy without triggering a crash.

MOVEMENT RATHER THAN EXERCISE

What differentiates movement from exercise? Exercise can be described as planned, structured, repetitive and intentional activity intended to improve or maintain physical fitness that may also raise the heart rate. It is guided by an external way of moving. As we slowly start to reconnect with all our levels of being through yoga and conscious breathing, however, we find we can move in positive ways that are very different from exercise. We become more attuned to internal sensations and how the external affects us. As we learn to feel into this, we begin to practise in ways that are more nourishing for our body. We can invite movement, together with breath and rest, and become curious as we explore, allow and pause.

LET'S PRACTISE: Creating space to breathe

This next practice, which can be done from sitting or lying, supports the idea that gentle awareness of breath and visualizing where the breath is can have a huge impact on our ability to create a sense of space.

1. Begin by noticing the parts of your body in contact with the surface you are on.

2. Take some time to gather a sense of stillness.

3. We are going to visualize bringing space to the joints of our body, using the breath. Visualization is a very powerful way of moving *prana* (energy) in the body, and in this way we can also help to free the joints. You can do the visualization and the physical practice, or just the visualization, depending on your energy levels. Start by focusing on your ankles and take three slow breaths here, visualizing space opening up in the ankle joints on each inhalation.

4. Begin to rotate each ankle, slowly one way and then the other. Continue to breathe and visualize space in this joint.

5. Next take three slow breaths to the knees, again visualizing space in the knee joints.

6. Begin to move, gently bending and flexing the knee joint, visualizing space as the knee moves.

7. Repeat with three slow breaths to the hips, wrists, elbows, shoulders and the jaw, all the time visualizing space coming into the joints with the breath. You can also move each joint in whatever way feels good for you.

8. Visualize your body full of space so that energy in the form of *prana* flows freely.

9. Lying quietly, you may like to set an intention: 'I let go of fear by being here in this present moment. I remember that in this moment there is nothing to fear. There is only fear if I leave this moment and this is just a thought.' Pause and notice the stillness and silence.

10. Contemplate these questions: 'How real are my thoughts? If they are always changing, am I my thoughts or something more?' and 'Can I meet myself with acceptance, just as I am right now?'

INCREASING ENERGY VIA THE BREATH

Many of the benefits of aerobic exercise are due to increased oxygenation at a cellular level. The good news is that we can use breathing practices in order to benefit the body and brain in the same way, without the danger of a relapse. In fact, yoga and breathing practices are a brilliant bio-hack!

LET'S PRACTISE: Slow moving, slow breathing

This practice encourages both the upper body muscles and the diaphragm to relax (vital for better breathing and better balance), and also helps to release the spine. Over time, you may wish to match the movements to a balanced, coherent (*samana*) breath, extending the inhale and exhale to an even rhythm (as detailed in Chapter 4).

1. Begin from a seated position on a chair, or sit comfortably on a yoga mat. You might

like to support your legs with cushions or experiment with other positions, such as leaning on a wall, or legs out in front with a cushion under the knees.

2. Imagine drawing a line up your spine, beginning from the tailbone to the crown of the head. It may help to visualize that you are creating space for your body to breathe as you lift your heart and ribs up slightly and relax your shoulders down away from your ears.

3. Inhale gently through the nose, visualizing the breath travelling up the spine.

4. Exhale, visualizing the breath releasing down the spine.

5. Continue to breathe slowly and gently through the nose, visualizing the breath moving up and down the spine.

6. Inhale. As you exhale, gently tilt your head to the right, bringing your right ear towards your right shoulder.

7. Stay here for a few breaths. Inhale, coming back to the centre, then exhale, and this time tilt your head to the left, bringing your left ear towards your left shoulder. Pause for a few breaths. Centre your head on an inhalation.

8. Repeat a few times, focusing on a slow, gentle breath. Now just sit quietly for a few breaths.

9. Roll your shoulders gently towards your ears on an inhale; as you exhale, let the shoulders release down. Continue to breathe in this way, imagining the shoulders moving further from the ears each time you exhale.

10. Roll the shoulders a few times more, continuing to breathe slowly and gently through the nose.

11. Come down to the floor into a Cat position, with your knees under your hips and your hands under your shoulders. Experiment with where to place your hands. It might be more comfortable to bring them slightly forward, with your weight over your hips. If it's more comfortable to stay seated, you can do the same movements, in which case rest your hands on your lap.

12. Stay in a neutral Cat position for a few breaths, focusing on space between the knees, feet, toes, shoulders, hands and fingers. Focus on creating space from the crown of your head to the tailbone.

13. If you are sitting, focus on the length of the spine and the space between the crown of the head and the tailbone as you gently lift the ribs.

14. From sitting, on the inhalation, lift your heart, feeling the front body open and the spine lengthen. If you are on the floor, lift the heart up as you breathe in.

15. Exhale and curl the chin to the chest arching the spine, taking the navel towards the spine. Repeat 3–5 times, or for as long as is comfortable, moving the spine in time with the breath, inhaling to lift the chest/heart and exhaling to round the spine. Over time, you can extend the inhale and the exhale to make the movement slower.

16. Rest in the chair or come down to lie comfortably. Focus on the feeling of your body in contact with the floor. Relax for a few breaths.

17. Come back to a Cat position if you are on the floor. If you wish to remain seated, then visualize the next movement. Slowly circle the pelvis, first one way and then the other. You can continue to circle your hips or experiment with the movement by making it bigger. Arch your spine, tuck your chin to chest, then rotate your hips and torso, as if your whole spine is a spoon stirring a pot. Notice areas of your back that need more attention and feel free to stay in one space for a few breaths, breathing gently into this area.

18. Continue to move in whatever way feels good for you for a few more breaths.

19. Rest in any way that feels comfortable for you – on your back or front.

FINDING BALANCE FOR BRAIN AND BODY

Balance is a complex system, and our ability to remain stable comes from three sensory inputs: the *vestibular system* (motion and spatial orientation), *vision* (eyesight) and *proprioception* (perception or awareness of the position and movement of the body). Practising balancing every day not only increases these skills, preventing falls and injuries, but also keeps our mind fit and mentally sharp, and helps us to navigate the ever-changing challenges of the world. This is especially important when we are recovering from an illness that may affect our cognition, focus and memory. Research shows that the ability to balance has positive effects on memory and spatial cognition (our ability to successfully understand, reason and remember location in our environment) (Rogge *et al.* 2017). We know the diaphragm is very important for our health in terms of breathing. New research demonstrates that the diaphragm is also vital for maintaining balance (Kocjan *et al.* 2018). Yoga and functional breathing are therefore very useful tools in maintaining and practising balance, because they connect all of these systems.

LET'S PRACTISE: Flamingo

The next practice is recognized as a functional age test (Cooper *et al.* 2014), and the results demonstrate that our ability to balance is a powerful predictor of longevity and health (Mosley 2022). Diaphragmatic breathing holds the key to balancing, together with fixing the gaze on a point of focus. Throughout the practice, breathe in a slow, low, steady way. Steady breath, steady body, steady mind!

Please use any support you need, such as holding the back of a chair or being near a wall. We include various options that you can use as your balance improves. As always, don't rush. Remember, this is not a test of endurance but an exploration of balancing.

Enjoy the journey as you channel your inner flamingo!

1. Begin from standing. Start in the posture known as *samasthiti*, which means standing in a balanced posture, feet hip width apart, ribs lifted, spine upright and shoulders relaxed. Feel the sensation of the floor under the feet, and have a sense of the feet spreading and widening. Your posture should feel alert, but also comfortable. Visualize your feet as solid on the floor. You might like to imagine they have roots going into the Earth beneath you, to help to give you balance.

2. Bringing awareness to your breath, place a hand on the belly, encouraging a slow, low breath through the nose.

3. Begin to shift your weight to the right foot, and slowly bring the left foot off the ground.

4. Remember, we progress through practice not perfection, and diaphragmatic breathing is a key to this posture, together with finding a point in front to focus your gaze on.

5. There are several alternative options for this pose, please choose the right one for you: (1) lift only the heel of the left foot off the ground, keeping the toes in contact with the floor; (2) lift the left foot and balance it on the instep of the right foot; (3) lift the left foot and, bending the left knee, bring it up to hip height; hold around the knee and bring it softly in towards the body; and (4) lifting the left foot, bend the knee downwards, bringing your foot up behind you to touch your buttock or towards the back of the thigh; hold around the foot.

6. As you balance on one leg, hold a chair or a wall if you need to. You might like to touch your support intermittently, so you know it is there. Allowing ourselves the support we need is an important part of self-care.

7. Continuing to focus on the breath and gazing at one point either on the floor or the wall in front of you, balance for as long as is comfortable. Notice how you respond to balancing in this posture. Bring awareness to any changes in the breath. Is it smooth, subtle, slow and low? Notice any sensations in the body such as wobbling (which is fine) and remember to stay within a place of comfort. This means that if you start to sway too much or if your muscles start to shake, please come out and rest.

8. Repeat on the other leg by lifting up the right foot in the same way as you did the left. Notice without judgement differences between the two sides of the body. We are not comparing or judging – we are not meant to be symmetrical – we carry ourselves, our lives and our belongings differently on each side, so you may find it easier to balance on one side than the other. You might like to progress towards holding for the same

length of time on both sides, so we introduce the concept of *samana* (balance) to the whole of our *panca maya* (our whole being).

9. Sit and rest or take time to lie down for a few minutes before going back into your day.

THE POWER OF VISUALIZATION

Another way that we can bring the benefits of exercise to our bodies at rest is by using guided visualization. Mental rehearsal, or visualization, has been used for many years in sports, by athletes, musicians and even chess grand masters. In a study by exercise psychologist Guang Yue, the results of those who exercised physically using finger movement were compared to those who only visualized moving their fingers. In the physical exercise group, finger abduction strength increased by 53 per cent (Ranganathan *et al.* 2004). In the group who only mentally rehearsed the muscle contractions, strength increased by 35 per cent. However, the greatest gain (40%) was seen four weeks after training had ceased in the group who visualized the movement (Ranganathan *et al.* 2004).

This study may only be about finger strength, but further studies on the brain activity in weightlifters showed similar effects. It was found that the muscles that were activated when a weightlifter lifted hundreds of pounds were similarly strengthened when they only visualized lifting. This demonstrates the incredible power of our minds. Interestingly, this correlates with what the ancient yogis claimed: where the mind goes, *prana* flows. Visualization is therefore a powerful tool in both science and yoga. The use of mental imagery impacts many processes in our brain such as perception, planning and memory. Combined with positive affirmation, we can use mental rehearsal and visualization to enhance the flow of *prana* within the whole body (*panca maya*). This can be especially useful if you are recovering from PoTs as you can visualize transitioning from different positions and this is why, throughout the book, we have included options to visualize any movement in case you are unable to physically do them.

WORKING WITH POTS

Many people with Long Covid and ME/CFS experience a form of dysautonomia known as Postural Orthostatic Tachycardia Syndrome (PoTS). PoTS can develop after a viral illness or traumatic event. The exact causes are still unclear, but we do know that symptoms of PoTS are often due to a sudden surge in heart rate as the body struggles to pump the blood back to the heart quickly enough. In response, blood vessels constrict and the pulse increases to maintain blood flow to the brain and heart to prevent blood pressure dropping. This can cause heart palpitations and feelings of faintness, especially when changing position from lying to sitting, or sitting to standing, and can also impact the ability to maintain concentration.

PoTS affects memory and is linked to a combination of symptoms including brain fog. This has implications for anyone teaching or practising yoga, as the changes in posture as we transition from one position to another, especially if done too quickly, often exaggerate symptoms, causing extreme dizziness. Therefore, we must encourage those with Long Covid to pause and rest rather than getting up too fast. We also need to keep our guidance during the practice very simple, without too much description, because many experience brain fog and exhaustion as a result of PoTS.

LET'S PRACTISE: The breath body wave

This practice invites visualization of breath and movement of the body like a wave on the ocean. You might like to combine the visualization with imagining the soothing sound of the sea.

1. Start from a lying position with knees bent and feet flat on the floor. Focus your attention on the parts of the body in contact with your support.

2. Notice the breath. Without judgement, observe the quality of the breath. Is it smooth or ragged? If the breath was a wave, would it be a gentle ripple of a wave on a calm sea, or something more choppy? Perhaps today the breath feels like a towering wall of water?

3. Place a hand on the belly and encourage the breath to become slow and low, envisaging the breath as a ripple of a wave coming into shore and back out again, like a gentle procession of shimmering peaks under the sun's soft glow.

4. Continue to breathe in this way as you allow the gentle rise and fall of the belly to connect to the image of the rhythmic waves, undulating in and out of the shoreline.

5. Bring your attention to your feet. Now lift the heels as you roll onto the balls of the feet as you breathe in, then back to the heels, as you breathe out, so the movement is in time with the inhale and exhale, the rise and fall of the wave on the shoreline.

6. Move this imagery of the waves up the body now towards the pelvis. Keeping the feet flat on the ground, begin to rock forwards and backwards, tilting the pelvis forwards with the inhale and back with the exhale. As you move forwards, the pelvis tilts and the lower arch of the back moves away from the ground. As you tilt the pelvis backwards, the lower back presses down into the ground.

7. You can continue with this movement, or begin to lift the spine gently off the ground with each inhale, slowly and gently allowing the waves of the breath to guide the movement of your body. With each inhale the hips slowly rise, and with each exhale the spine slowly makes its way back down to the ground.

8. Listen and be kind to your energy levels. You don't need to lift too high or to do too many repetitions. Remember to practise with kindness to self, and always with comfort in mind.

9. Continue with this movement for a few more breaths.

10. Come back and rest with the knees bent, observing the movement of the breath for a few moments.

11. Keeping the back on the support, let the arms float up and through the air with every wave of breath guiding the movement of the body. They may just lift a little, or they may come up and back towards the floor behind your head. Just do this a few times, listening to your body and honouring your energy levels.

12. Rest, with the palms down by the hips, for a few moments and explore how you feel. Mind, body, breath, emotions and energy.

13. If your energy is still all right, you may wish to now combine the movement of the arms with the movement of the hips lifting, as you move in and out of a very gentle bridge position. Please remember there is no need to force anything or to feel discomfort. Every movement is a choice and you can rest any time or modify to a simpler movement that is easier for you, at any time.

14. Continue for a few more breaths. Then gently rest, so the arms are beside the hips, palms down. Bring awareness back to the sensation of the body being in contact with the ground.

15. Hug the knees towards the chest and rock from side to side.

16. Finding a sense of space, make yourself comfortable and settle into rest.

THE IMPORTANCE OF PLAY FOR WELLBEING

In many ways, allowing ourselves to move freely or to use our imagination in the way that yoga encourages can feel like playing. Reconnecting to our innate sense of playfulness can in itself be a wonderful healing practice, and encouraging playful activities is a well-researched way of improving mood, reducing stress and increasing overall wellbeing. It's important to note that many of the practices in the book are useful for children, too. Although our next chapter focuses specifically on practices for children recovering from Long Covid, they are just as useful for adults.

KEY POINTS

✓ National Institute for Health and Care Excellence (NICE) guidelines make it clear that incorporating incremental increases in physical activity is not suitable for individuals with fatigue-based conditions.

✓ Some medical professionals continue to encourage exercise as treatment, resulting in relapse.

✓ Post-exertional malaise (PEM) refers to the worsening of symptoms and fatigue following physical, emotional or cognitive exertion.

✓ Pacing is vital to ensure recovery from fatigue-based illness.

✓ Reframing our relationship to exercise can be difficult, as physical exercise is often used to manage and support mental health.

✓ Slowing down can be difficult if we are used to living at a fast pace or with a chronic stress response.

✓ Movement rather than exercise is key. Slow, mindful movement allows us to move in ways that nourish rather than punish the body.

✓ Breathing well can increase energy at a cellular level.

✓ Diaphragmatic breathing helps our ability to find balance in our minds and bodies.

✓ Visualization and mental imagery techniques have been used for years to rehearse movement and improve performance.

✓ Using imagination and play can increase feelings of wellbeing, and is vital for recovery.

Chapter 12

NURTURING RECOVERY

A Guide for Children Recovering from Long Covid

NADYNE MCKIE

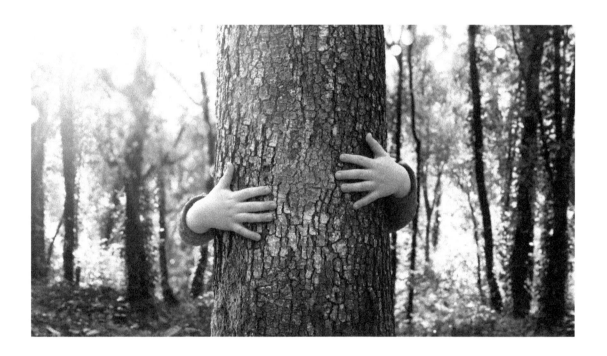

I feel well placed to write this chapter as my son suffered with fatigue for over a year following a Covid-19 infection. It is heartbreaking to see your child transform from an energetic, life-loving young person to one who can barely stand for long periods, can't focus on schoolwork, and who becomes unable to take part in their normal activities. We were lucky to have a fantastic paediatric consultant, who understood the dangers of post-viral fatigue in young people. In this chapter I share the guidance he gave that helped us support our son to recuperate and recover, along with child-friendly yoga and breathing practices that helped with his healing.

For a child with Long Covid, their experience might involve symptoms such as persistent fatigue, breathing difficulties, muscle and joint pain, headaches and brain fog.

Normal everyday activities become challenging, and they need to rest frequently. School attendance may suffer and social interactions become limited, leading to feelings of isolation. Recovery can be slow, requiring patience and support from family, friends, school and healthcare professionals. Nobody wants to see their child suffer in this way and so, as parents and caregivers, we may push our children to try to get better quickly so they can resume their daily lives. But pressures on parents to work, care for other children and go about their own daily lives impact upon the child's recovery. The logistical 'inconvenience' of having a child off school can be very challenging for parents, and yet, we must learn to listen to our young people and respond with compassion, empathy and care. If we don't, the resulting detrimental effects are evident throughout this book:

> The memory that stands out most for me was taking my son to see the paediatrician in London. The train journey, taxi ride to the hospital and then the actual appointment meant that by 11am my son was fast asleep on a couch in a coffee shop. He was totally worn out, with no energy even to talk, let alone drink his hot chocolate. It really hit me then that my child's fatigue was a very real and very misunderstood symptom. To see my son unable to function normally was heartbreaking.

It's essential to approach recovery from Long Covid with patience, positivity and the right strategies. Long Covid can be debilitating, and the recovery journey can be isolating. Overly focusing on what has been lost, and what may be being missed out on, can drive feelings of hopelessness and despair, further affecting the nervous system, and impacting the mental health of both the child and the parent/carer. Acceptance of what is, on each day, can be a useful way to manage these feelings. This involves awareness that each day is different, with compassion for whatever arises. Spend time focusing on what your child is still able to participate in, set realistic achievable goals and celebrate the wins that each day brings with gratitude, no matter how small!

This chapter is focused on guiding you through the process of incorporating yoga practices suitable for children, fostering functional breathing and effectively communicating your needs to your child's school, who may not be aware of the need for pacing, rest and gradual recovery from post-viral symptoms.

Generally, children are better able to listen to their body signals and communicate to us what they are feeling. It's very important, however, that we listen and that we give them recognition and validation. Recently on social media, a prominent psychologist asked for stories from people whose experience had been disbelieved when they were young. The psychologist wanted to know how this had affected them. There were many who recounted experiences of feeling unwell, that were dismissed by caregivers. The long-term effects and trauma of this are reflected in this book. When the ability to listen to what the body is saying is dismissed, and the child learns that they need to ignore, disconnect and repress their physical and emotional symptoms, this has very negative consequences. As adults we then become adept at ignoring our signals in order to carry on and push on through. This book offers an opportunity to change this pattern.

Clearly, supporting a child as they recover places additional demands upon parents. Children need plenty of fluids, good nutrition, adequate sleep and rest, rest, rest. This is not easy when we are used to seeing our child full of energy and life, because this, of course, affects our own wellbeing too. We may have sleepless nights, not be able to take enough down-time to rest, and not be eating good nutritious food, because we may feel there is no time to prioritize our own health. It's therefore vital to seek as much support for yourself as you can over this time.

EMBRACING HEALING YOGA PRACTICES FOR CHILDREN

Yoga can be a wonderful tool to support a child's recovery. Engaging in simple, child-friendly poses that promote relaxation, flexibility and inner balance can assist in resetting the nervous system, which can be dysregulated following viral infection. Many of the practices in the book are suitable for children, and just like adults, even when we are used to living very active lifestyles, we must focus on encouraging children to move much more gently during recovery from Long Covid. A dynamic yoga practice is not the best way to begin yoga for children. Instead, we suggest simple movements focused on grounding, playful postures and rest.

However, with breath-based practices it is not advisable to attempt balanced breathing using a 5–6 second count for inhale/exhale, as children's lungs do not have the same capacity as adults.

FUNCTIONAL BREATHING FOR CHILDREN

As we know from previous chapters, functional breathing involves using the diaphragm to breathe low and slow through the nose, promoting relaxation and efficient oxygenation into the body. It's important for children to understand that breathing well supports their health, emotions and concentration.

Children naturally breathe diaphragmatically when they are babies, but life events and illness can create poor breathing patterns, even at a young age. Mouth breathing is a known risk factor in many health conditions affecting children such as behavioural issues, anxiety, asthma and chronic illness (Kalaskar *et al.* 2021).

It's important to work slowly and gently with this age group as we guide them towards a better breathing pattern that includes nasal breathing. The benefits of working with children are that we can approach healing using creative and imaginative tools and practices. You may wish to begin by using the 'Drawing the breath' practice, as described in Chapter 3.

LET'S PRACTISE: Breath awareness game

1. Introduce the idea of becoming aware of the breath.

2. Offer reassurance that it is normal for us to not notice our breathing, but this game is about focusing on how we breathe.

3. Set a timer for 1 minute. The invitation is to sit or lie quietly, paying attention to the breath without trying to change it.

4. After the 1 minute, chat with the child about what they noticed.

5. How fast was their breathing?

6. Where did the breath go when they inhaled? What part of the body moved most?

7. Was the breath steady and smooth, or did it feel bumpy?

8. Was the inhale longer or shorter than the exhale?

9. As we become more attuned with the breath, we can pose these questions as we breathe as a way to encourage slower, smoother breathing.

LET'S PRACTISE: Balloon breathing for releasing anxiety

Encouraging slow, diaphragmatic breathing for children is an essential practice for recovery.

1. Sitting or lying comfortably, focus on breathing through the nose.

2. Gradually begin to slow the breath down by placing a hand on the belly. We are going to imagine blowing up a balloon in your tummy.

3. On each inhale, the balloon becomes bigger and inflates and the belly rises.

4. On each exhale, the balloon slowly deflates and the belly releases.

5. Repeat a few times, until feeling calm and centred.

LET'S PRACTISE: Breathing in nature

For children with fatigue and Long Covid symptoms, time outside may be limited due to lack of energy. However, it's important that children get outside when possible. We know that nature is healing. Even in inner cities, we can find pockets of peace and calm in green spaces. If possible, encourage them to stand barefoot on the earth if it is warm enough and if you have access to outside space. This helps them to feel grounded and connected. The invitation of this practice is to encourage connection to the breath as a way to connect to the natural world around us.

1. Go outdoors and find a peaceful, quiet spot.

2. Sitting or standing in one place, notice how it feels to have your feet in contact with the ground.

3. Notice if any parts of the body feel tight or tense.

4. Inhale and imagine breathing in the fresh air.

5. As you exhale, imagine releasing any feelings of tightness or tension into the air.

6. You may like to imagine breathing in the colours around you, the blue sky, the green grass, perhaps a coloured flower or leaf.

7. Take time to rest and chat about the experience of breathing in nature.

LET'S PRACTISE: Rainbow bubbles – breathing to release anxiety

Illness and social isolation can result in anxiety for children. They may fear being unwell, relapsing and missing out on time with friends and participating in usual activities. Connecting to the present moment and encouraging children to take each day at a time can be helpful in reducing anxiety. Co-regulation is key when we are looking after our children. Take time to care for yourself too – this is very important – so that you feel grounded and calm before practising with your child. Remember, your state of mind will affect your child too, so self-care is vital.

1. Lying or sitting comfortably, find a space where you feel as comfortable as you can be.

2. Let's begin to connect to the breath. Notice the inhale and the exhale.

3. We are going to imagine blowing bubbles. You can place any worries inside the bubble and send the worries up, up and away.

4. Imagine the colours of the rainbow: red, orange, yellow, green, blue, indigo, violet. You may wish to add your own favourite colour. Each bubble can be a colour, if you like that idea.

5. Inhale, and imagine the bubble and the worry you wish to place inside it; as you exhale, blow into the bubble and see the colour of the bubble with the worry inside.

6. As you breathe out, imagine it drifting up, up and away.

7. Take a breath in between each bubble. You might even like to try this with a real bubble wand.

8. Keep blowing bubbles for as long as you need.

9. Rest for a while.

YOGA AND MEDITATION FOR CHILDREN

Many of the practices in this book are suitable for children, and, just like adults, even when we are used to living very active lifestyles, we must focus on encouraging children to move much more gently during recovery from Long Covid. A dynamic yoga practice is not the best way to begin yoga for children. Instead, we suggest simple movements focused on grounding, playful postures and rest.

LET'S PRACTISE: Rainbow meditation

Using colours can give a focus to meditation for children. This practice encourages slow, gentle breathing and rest.

1. Take time to make yourself as comfortable as possible.

2. Close your eyes, and notice how your body feels when it's in a comfy space.

3. Placing a hand on your tummy, notice if you can slow your breathing down so you feel the hand on the tummy softly rising and falling with each breath. If this is not possible today, it's okay, just focus on each breath as you breathe in and out.

4. Imagine you are walking down a path. It's been lightly raining, but now the sun is shining and in the distance you see a beautiful rainbow.

5. Stand under the rainbow and let yourself see all the colours and the warm, bright light.

6. With each colour repeat the following phrases:

   - Red: I am strong.

   - Orange: I am playful.

   - Yellow: I am kind.

   - Green: I am caring.

   - Blue: I am honest.

   - Indigo: I am creative.

   - Violet: I am safe.

7. You can continue to breathe in this way and repeat the phrases as many times as you like. Remember, if one of the phrases feels tricky to say to yourself, you can let yourself notice this without any judgement or you can change the phrase to something that feels just right for you.

8. Let yourself stay in this comfy space for as long as you need, under this rainbow, where the colours shine brightly upon you.

COMMUNICATING YOUR CHILD'S NEEDS

Many adults with Long Covid may have experienced trying to communicate symptoms to doctors and other healthcare professionals, only to be dismissed. When caring for a child who is recovering, we must learn to advocate for them. Communication with schools is a key part of this process. Like many chronic conditions, Long Covid is an invisible illness, and when a child appears fine to others, this can reinforce dismissal of symptoms and be perceived as school refusal or anxiety.

School is an essential part of our children's lives. Education and social skills suffer when children are absent, and there is often immense pressure upon schools and parents to ensure that the child attend as much as they can. At the beginning of the chapter, I mentioned my son's paediatrician who was excellent in assisting us in communicating the risks involved in placing pressure upon a child to take part in activities that might impact healing and recovery. Here are some useful tips and guidance on how to inform and communicate a child's needs to their school:

- A gradual return to normal activities is the best way. Do not force a child to maintain daily activities if they are unable to. As adults, we know we should not be exercising and working if we are chronically unwell ourselves, and we must learn to care for our children in the same way if we want longer-term recovery.

- Arrange a meeting with the school to discuss a gradual flexible return. Seeking support from specialist medical professionals, educational psychologists, special educational needs coordinators (SENCos) and occupational therapists can be a useful way to reinforce and give support in best informing the school as to your child's needs at this time.

- If a child is able to attend school, it is often best that they do so for mornings or afternoons and not for the full day, as this can leave them depleted and exhausted, resulting in relapse and further time away. It is better that they attend for the small period of time that they are able to cope with, rather than being forced to be in school for a full day, resulting in relapse.

- Encourage doing less, even when the child thinks they can do more. Physical activities can be exhausting for children with Long Covid and fatigue. Communicate that pacing is required and that there is a very real danger of relapse if they are pushed to join in sports and PE. Post-exertional malaise (PEM) is a well-known symptom of fatigue. The need for rest is a priority. It must be a non-pressure-based approach to assessing whether a child is able to join in PE lessons, and our advice is to take time away from sports and PE until a child is easily able to attend three to four days at school without relapse. Our paediatrician advised that it was essential to be able to achieve activities without being fatigued, because over-exertion will put the child in a worse position for recovery.

- Cardiac screening may be required before returning to sports. Seek medical advice.

- Fatigue is not just about physical activities. We know that our brain uses a vast amount of energy. Learning new things can be exhausting for a child with fatigue. Breaking up tasks into smaller chunks of time can be useful as well as encouraging children to rest after learning. This especially means time away from screens, as they erode and deplete energy levels, and can tax an already dysregulated nervous system. This includes TV watching. Screens and TV are tempting because they may temporarily numb symptoms. However, they also disconnect the body from cues of when to stop or when there is exhaustion. Therefore, screentime should ideally be minimized.

- Ensure your child can sustain improvements for a period of time before increasing any activity. This is especially the case with children, who will naturally want to join in activities that they feel they are missing out on, and so may be encouraged, or force themselves, to do more than their bodies are able to.

- Build in as much rest time as you would activities. Plan for as much rest as possible.

- Start small. Just a few minutes of concentration may be possible at first. This is okay. Slowly and gradually is the best way. Work with your child to consider energy levels required for different activities. You might like to categorize them into low, medium and high energy.

- Social interaction is an essential part of a child's life; however, like adults, being around lots of people for long periods of time can be exhausting. Noise can be overwhelming when dealing with Long Covid symptoms, and so limiting time in noisy environments is part of the process of managing recovery.

We know how difficult it can be to manage convalescence for ourselves, and so managing our child's recovery in a society that enforces lack of agency in children, dismisses children's needs and often encourages repression of feelings ('don't cry', 'man up', 'you can do it if you try hard enough', etc.) is not conducive to healing. In a society where children are so often judged on results and performance, the inability to participate and achieve in school and activities due to illness can be incredibly impactful on mental health. We must advocate for and support our children as we navigate the recovery journey with them.

Advocating for our children means empowering ourselves with information and educating others when they may have strongly held opinions. This can all be overwhelming. *It's vital for caregivers and parents to take time to look after themselves in this process.* We can often become the last priority when it comes to caring for others, but it is indeed a vital part of the recovery journey, and you will be better able to manage if you are well supported and rested yourself. The practices in this book are a helpful resource for caregivers, and we invite you to use them as a tool for your own self-care if you are caring for others.

KEY POINTS

- ✓ Caring for children who are unwell and unable to attend school, or function as they once did in daily life, requires that we support ourselves as parents and carers with the same attention as our children.

- ✓ This can feel very demanding due to work, family and the additional pressure of advocating for our child with fatigue.

- ✓ Isolation from friends may encourage more time online. Screentime, however, can add to dysfunctional breathing patterns and increase feelings of anxiety.

- ✓ Simple practices that cultivate and encourage calm and creativity can help children to breathe better and to rest in ways that allow the body to replenish and recover.

References

Akaberi, D., Krambrich, J., Ling, J., Luni, C., *et al.* (2020) 'Mitigation of the replication of SARS-CoV-2 by nitric oxide in vitro.' *Redox Biology 37*, 101734. www.sciencedirect.com/science/article/pii/S2213231720309393

Balban, M.Y., Neri, E., Kogon, M.M., Weed, L., *et al.* (2023) 'Brief structured respiration practices enhance mood and reduce physiological arousal.' *Cell Reports. Medicine 4*, 1, 100895. doi: 10.1016/j.xcrm.2022.100895.

Bayer, L., Constantinescu, I., Perrig, S., Vienne, J., *et al.* (2011) 'Rocking synchronizes brain waves during a short nap.' *Current Biology 21*, 12, R461–R462. https://doi.org/10.1016/j.cub.2011.05.012

Brown, R.P. and Gerbarg, P.L. (2012) *The Healing Power of the Breath: Simple Techniques to Reduce Stress and Anxiety, Enhance Concentration, and Balance Your Emotions*. Boston, MA: Trumpeter.

Cooper, R., Strand, B.H., Hardy, R., Patel, K.V. and Kuh, D. (2014) 'Physical capability in mid-life and survival over 13 years of follow-up: British birth cohort study.' *The BMJ 348*. https://doi.org/10.1136/bmj.g2219

Cottle, M.H. (1987) 'The work, ways, positions and patterns of nasal breathing (relevance in heart and lung illness).' [Reprinted in Strohl, K.P., Arnold, J.L., Hoekje, P.L. and McFadden, E.R. (1992) 'Nasal flow-resistive responses to challenge with cold dry air.' *Journal of Applied Physiology 72*, 4, 1243–1246. doi: 10.1152/jappl.1992.72.4.1243.]

Cox, D. (2022) 'Can our mitochondria help to beat Long Covid?' *The Observer*, 26 June. www.theguardian.com/science/2022/jun/26/can-our-mitochondria-help-to-beat-long-covid

Dallam, G.M., McClaran, S.R., Cox, D.G. and Foust, C.P. (2018) 'Effect of nasal versus oral breathing on Vo2max and physiological economy in recreational runners following an extended period spent using nasally restricted breathing.' *International Journal of Kinesiology and Sports Science 6*, 2, 22–29. doi: 10.7575/aiac.ijkss.v.6n.2p.22.

Dana, D. (2018) *The Polyvagal Theory in Therapy: Engaging the Rhythm of Regulation*. Norton Series on Interpersonal Neurobiology. New York: W.W. Norton & Co.

Desikachar, T.K.V. (1999) *The Heart of Yoga: Developing a Personal Practice* (2nd edn). Rochester, VT: Inner Traditions.

Desikachar, T.K.V. (2003) *Reflections on Yoga Sutras of Patanjali (Revised edition)*. Chennai, India: Krishnamacharya Yoga Mandiram.

Drew, L. (2023) 'Why relaxation is as important as sleep – and six ways to do it better.' *New Scientist*, 30 August. www.newscientist.com/article/mg25934540-800-why-relaxation-is-as-important-as-sleep-and-six-ways-to-do-it-better

Felitti, V.J., Anda, R.F., Nordenberg, D., Williamson, D.F., *et al.* (1998) 'Relationship of childhood abuse and household dysfunction to many of the leading causes of death in adults: The Adverse Childhood Experiences (ACE) Study.' *American Journal of Preventive Medicine 14*, 4, 245–258. https://doi.org/10.1016/S0749-3797(98)00017-8

Feuerstein, G. (1990) *Encyclopedic Dictionary of Yoga*. Unwin Health. London: Unwin Paperbacks.

Geller, S.M. and Porges, S.W. (2014) 'Therapeutic presence: Neurophysiological mechanisms mediating feeling safe in therapeutic relationships.' *Journal of Psychotherapy Integration 24*, 3, 178–192. https://doi.org/10.1037/a0037511

Germain, A., Ruppert, D., Levine, S.N. and Hampson, M.R. (2018) 'Prospective biomarkers from plasma metabolomics of Myalgic Encephalomyelitis/Chronic Fatigue Syndrome implicate redox imbalance in disease symptomatology.' *Metabolites* 8, 4, 90. doi: 10.3390/metabo8040090.

Granger, T. (2019) *Draw Breath: The Art of Breathing, Mindfulness & Meditation.* London: Vie Books.

Grey, D.B. (2019) *Quantum Physics Made Easy: The Introduction Guide for Beginners Who Flunked Maths and Science in Plain Simple English.* Independently published.

Gupta, A.H. (2023) 'Checking email? You're probably not breathing.' *The New York Times*, 21 August. www.nytimes.com/2023/08/21/well/live/screen-apnea-breathing.html

Hammond, C. and Lewis, G. (2016) 'The Rest Test: Preliminary Findings from a Large-Scale International Survey on Rest.' In F. Callard, K. Staines and J. Wilkes (eds) *The Restless Compendium: Interdisciplinary Investigations of Rest and Its Opposites* (Chapter 8). Basingstoke: Palgrave Macmillan. www.ncbi.nlm.nih.gov/books/NBK453237

Hanson, R. (2013) *Hardwiring Happiness: The Practical Science of Reshaping Your Brain.* London: Rider Books.

Hanson, R. and Mendius, R. (2009) *Buddha's Brain: The Practical Neuroscience of Happiness, Love & Wisdom.* Oakland, CA: New Harbinger Publications Inc.

Heim, C., Nater, U.M., Maloney, E., Boneva, R., Jones, J.F. and Reeves, W.C. (2009) 'Childhood trauma and risk for chronic fatigue syndrome.' *Archives of General Psychiatry* 66, 1, 72–80. doi: 10.1001/archgenpsychiatry.2008.508.

Kalaskar, R., Bhaje, P., Kalaskar, A. and Faye, A. (2021) 'Sleep difficulties and symptoms of attention-deficit hyperactivity disorder in children with mouth breathing.' *International Journal of Clinical Pediatric Dentistry* 14, 5, 604–609. doi: 10.5005/jp-journals-10005-1987.

Kocjan, J., Gzik-Zroska, B., Nowakowska, K., Burkacki, M., *et al.* (2018) 'Impact of diaphragm function parameters on balance maintenance.' *PLoS ONE* 13, 12, e0208697. https://doi.org/10.1371/journal.pone.0208697

Levine, P.A. (2008) *Healing Trauma: A Pioneering Program for Restoring the Wisdom of Your Body.* Louisville, CO: Sounds True.

Mancini, D., Brunjes, D., Lala, A., Trivieri, M.G., Contreras, J.P. and Natelson, B.H. (2021) 'Use of cardiopulmonary stress testing for patients with unexplained dyspnea post-coronavirus disease.' *JACC: Journal of the American College of Cardiology: Heart Failure* 9, 12, 927–937. https://doi.org/10.1016/j.jchf.2021.10.002

Maté, G. (with Maté, D.) (2022) *The Myth of Normal: Trauma, Illness and Healing in a Toxic Culture.* London: Vermilion.

McKeown, P. (2015) *The Oxygen Advantage: Simple, Scientifically Proven Breathing Technique to Help You Become Healthier, Slimmer, Faster, and Fitter.* New York: William Morrow & Company.

Mosley, M. (2022) 'Take the balance challenge to help you live longer.' BBC Science Focus, 1 March. www.sciencefocus.com/the-human-body/dr-michael-mosley-standing-on-one-leg

Naviaux, R.K., Naviaux, J.C., Li, K., Bright, A.T., *et al.* (2016) 'Metabolic features of chronic fatigue syndrome.' *PNAS: Proceedings of the National Academy of Sciences of the United States of America* 113, 37, E5472–E5480. doi: 10.1073/pnas.1607571113.

NHS CUH (Cambridge University Hospitals) (2019) 'Breathing control advice.' www.cuh.nhs.uk/patient-information/breathing-control-advice

NICE (National Institute for Health and Care Excellence) (2021) 'Myalgic encephalomyelitis (or encephalopathy)/chronic fatigue syndrome: Diagnosis and management.' NICE Guideline [NG206]. www.nice.org.uk/guidance/ng206

NICE (2021) 'NICE ME/CFS guideline outlines steps for better diagnosis and management.' News, 28 October. www.nice.org.uk/news/article/nice-me-cfs-guideline-outlines-steps-for-better-diagnosis-and-management

ONS (Office for National Statistics) (2023) 'Prevalence of ongoing symptoms following coronavirus (COVID-19) infection in the UK: 30 March 2023.' Data and analysis from Census 2021. Health and social care. www.ons.gov.uk/peoplepopulationandcommunity/healthandsocialcare/conditionsanddiseases/bulletins/prevalenceofongoingsymptomsfollowingcoronaviruscovid19infectionintheuk/30march2023

Outhoff, K. (2020) 'Sick and tired of COVID-19: Long haulers and post viral (fatigue) syndromes.' *South African General Practitioner* 1, 4, 132–134. doi: 10.36303/SAGP.2020.1.4.0041.

Porges, S.W. (2011) *The Polyvagal Theory: Neurophysiological Foundations of Emotions, Attachment, Communication, and Self-Regulation.* New York: W.W. Norton & Co.

Prior, R. (2021) 'A Stanford scientist's quest to cure his son could help unravel the mystery of Covid-19 long haulers.' CNN, 12 March. https://edition.cnn.com/2021/03/12/health/ron-davis-covid-long-hauler-scn-wellness/index.html

Ranganathan, V.K., Siemionow, V., Liu, J.Z., Sahgal, V. and Yue, G.H. (2004) 'From mental power to muscle power: Gaining strength by using the mind.' *Neuropsychologia* 42, 7, 944–956. doi: 10.1016/j.neuropsychologia.2003.11.018.

Rogge, A.K., Röder, B., Zech, A., Nagel, V., *et al.* (2017) 'Balance training improves memory and spatial cognition in healthy adults.' *Scientific Reports* 7, 1, 5661. doi: 10.1038/s41598-017-06071-9.

Rothenberg, R. (2019) *Restoring Prana: A Therapeutic Guide to Pranayama and Healing Through the Breath for Yoga Therapists, Yoga Teachers and Healthcare Practitioners.* London: Singing Dragon.

Spotila, J. (2010) 'Post-Exertional Malaise in Chronic Fatigue Syndrome.' Charlotte, NC: The CFIDS Association of America. https://solvecfs.org/wp-content/uploads/2013/10/pem-series.pdf

Steffen, P.R., Bartlett, D., Channell, R.M., Jackman, K., *et al.* (2021) 'Integrating breathing techniques into psychotherapy to improve HRV: Which approach is best?' *Frontiers in Psychology* 12, 624254. doi: 10.3389/fpsyg.2021.624254.

Sud, S., Friedrich, J.O., Adhikari, N.K., Taccone, P., *et al.* (2014) 'Effect of prone positioning during mechanical ventilation on mortality among patients with acute respiratory distress syndrome: A systematic review and meta-analysis.' *CMAJ: Canadian Medical Association Journal* 186, 10, E381–E390. www.ncbi.nlm.nih.gov/pmc/articles/PMC4081236

Summer, J. and Rehman, A. (2024) 'Mouth taping for sleep: Does it work?' Sleep Foundation, 2 January. www.sleepfoundation.org/snoring/mouth-taping-for-sleep

Svensson, S., Olin, A.C. and Hellgren, J. (2006) 'Increased net water loss by oral compared to nasal expiration in healthy subjects.' *Rhinology* 44, 1, 74–77. PMID: 16550955.

Taneja, M.K. (2020) 'Modified Bhramari Pranayama in Covid 19 infection.' *Indian Journal of Otolaryngology and Head and Neck Surgery* 72, 3, 395–397. doi: 10.1007/s12070-020-01883-0.

Valk, S.L., Bernhardt, B.C., Trautwein, F.M., Böckler, A., *et al.* (2017) 'Structural plasticity of the social brain: Differential change after socio-affective and cognitive mental training.' *Science Advances* 3, 10:e1700489. doi: 10.1126/sciadv.1700489.

Van Den Hurk, A.W., Ujvari, C., Greenspan, N., Malaspina, D., Jimenez, X.F. and Walsh-Messinger, J. (2022) 'Childhood trauma exposure increases long covid risk.' [Preprint.] doi: 10.1101/2022.02.18.22271191.

van der Kolk, B.A. (1997) 'The psychobiology of posttraumatic stress disorder.' *The Journal of Clinical Psychiatry* 58, Suppl. 9, 16–24. PMID: 9329447.

van der Kolk, B.A. (2015) *The Body Keeps the Score: Mind, Brain and Body in the Transformation of Trauma.* Harmondsworth: Penguin Books.

Vink, M. and Vink-Niese, A. (2022) 'The updated NICE guidance exposed the serious flaws in CBT and graded exercise therapy trials for ME/CFS.' *Healthcare (Basel)* 10, 5, 898. doi: 10.3390/healthcare10050898.

WHO (World Health Organization) (2023) *Clinical Management of Covid-19: Living Guideline.* Geneva: WHO. www.who.int/publications/i/item/WHO-2019-nCoV-clinical-2023.2

Further Resources

Restful Yoga for Fatigue with Fiona Agombar, for details of online classes, retreats, the Facebook group Restful Yoga for Fatigue with Fiona and YouTube channel: www. fionaagombar.co.uk

Please visit Mindful Movement Method (www.mindfulmovementmethod.com and www. andbreathe.com) for further details of courses, how to work with Nadyne and social media links.

Long Covid Kids & Friends represent children and young people living with Long Covid and related illnesses, and the parents and caregivers who look after them: www. longcovidkids.org

Fiona and Nadyne are planning to set up a YouTube channel – please visit our websites for updates (www.fionaagombar.co.uk and https://themindedinstitute.com/profile/ nadyne-mckie).

Helen Lynam is a recommended nutritionist specializing in nutrition for those with Long Covid: www.cpd-uk.com/about-us/helen-lynam

There are many good podcasts, but we particularly recommend the 'Long Covid' podcast with Jackie Baxter (www.longcovidpodcast.com) and also Anna Grear, 'The Fatigue Files', HypnoCatalyst, available on most platforms including Spotify and Apple.

Index